Clinical Cases in LAA Occlusion

Martin W. Bergmann • Apostolos Tzikas
Nina C. Wunderlich

Clinical Cases in LAA Occlusion

Indication, Techniques, Devices, Implantation

Springer

Martin W. Bergmann
Standort Wandsbek
Cardiologicum Hamburg
Hamburg
Germany

Nina C. Wunderlich
Kardiovaskuläres Zentrum Darmstadt
Darmstadt
Germany

Apostolos Tzikas
AHEPA University Hospital
Interbalkan European Medical Center
Thessaloniki
Greece

ISBN 978-3-319-51429-1 ISBN 978-3-319-51431-4 (eBook)
DOI 10.1007/978-3-319-51431-4

Library of Congress Control Number: 2017939628

Printed on acid-free paper

This Springer imprint is published by Springer Nature
The registered company is Springer International Publishing AG
The registered company address is: Gewerbestrasse 11, 6330 Cham, Switzerland

Contents

Acknowledgments

We acknowledge the contribution of the following authors:

Jennifer Franke Department of Cardiology, University of Heidelberg, Heidelberg, Germany

Siew Yen Ho Cardiac Morphology Unit, Royal Brompton Hospital, London, England

Robert James Siegel The Heart Institute, Cedars-Sinai Medical Center, Los Angeles, California, USA

Kevin P. Walsh Mater Misericordiae University Hospital, Dublin, Ireland

Chapter 1
Background: Stroke Prevention in Patients with Atrial Fibrillation

1.1 Rationale for LAA Closure in 2017: Background

When starting or expanding a LAA closure program, the imminent question certainly raised by referring physicians, and possibly even by some patients, is: why go for a potentially risky cardiac intervention if a well proven drug therapy like NOAC is available? Many patients prefer a single 2–3 days hospital stay with a low risk cardiac intervention similar to pulmonary vein isolation or PFO closure, over a long-term therapy which increases sensitivity to skin bruises, gastro-intestinal bleeding and other side effects. Non-interventional general practitioners or other colleagues not close to the field may argue that evidence is not sufficient as the number of patients included in prospective trials is low and only available for the Watchman device. Randomized trials and prospective registries in over 500,000 patients treated with NOAC's are available. In the absence of a randomized trial comparing NOAC therapy to LAA closure, in-depth discussion of the available data is necessary to achieve consensus. This chapter focusses on a critical appraisal of NOAC study data and provides a simple algorithm incorporating both US and European guidelines regarding indication for LAA closure.

1.2 Stroke Prevention in Patients with Atrial Fibrillation: Role of Pulmonary Vein Isolation

Atrial fibrillation (AF), regardless if paroxysmal, persistent, long-standing persistent or permanent, confers a five-fold risk of stroke overall 5 times higher than in patients without atrial fibrillation. Individual risk is calculated on the basis of the CHA_2DS_2_VASc score with a score ≥1 indicating the need for oral anticoagulation; this means that, aside from younger (<65 years) patients without cardiovascular risk

M.W. Bergmann et al., *Clinical Cases in LAA Occlusion*,
DOI 10.1007/978-3-319-51431-4_1

factors, all patients with AF should receive a therapeutic measure for stroke prevention. CHA_2DS_2_VASc score calculators are available in many smartphone APP's and should be documented in every AF patient. From a European perspective, $CHADS_2$ is no longer in use. Patients with lone atrial fibrillation are often symptomatic even on one or more drugs meant for rhythm control. These patients will likely be eligible for pulmonary vein isolation (PVI) [1]. However, according to the guidelines and published data, the indication for oral anticoagulation even after PVI is strictly linked to the CHA_2DS_2_VASc score as the current interpretation of the effect of PVI in most patients is to convert symptomatic AF to asymptomatic AF. Whereas PVI reduces the burden of AF more efficiently than available drug therapies (i.e. from 3.6 to 0.3 h per day in one study), only 21% of patients were completely free of any AF episode during a follow up of 41.4 ± 15.1 months employing an implantable monitoring device. AF may also reoccur after long-lasting (>1 year) episode-free intervals [2]. Nonetheless, patients with a CHA_2DS_2_VASc of ≤1 were found to have a lower risk of stroke after PVI [3]. In summary, PVI is the treatment of choice in patients younger than 65 with no comorbidities. If successful, no long term oral anticoagulation is required. The majority of patients with a history of AF are in need of a life-long therapeutic strategy for stroke prevention independent of the treatment strategy chosen for AF itself, including PVI. Unlike the treatment of other medical conditions like hypertension, stroke prevention needs to be more aggressive and intense with increasing age, as the risk of stroke and clinical impact of a stroke increases.

1.3 Reality of Oral Anticoagulation in 2017

Although the guidelines recommend oral anticoagulation with warfarin in patients with AF and a $CHADS_2$ score >1 for many years, many patients still do not receive adequate stroke prevention. The Canadian stroke network found that 90% of patients admitted to their stroke units with known atrial fibrillation and no known contraindication for anticoagulation were not receiving adequate medical stroke prevention: 29% presented with an INR <2, 29% were on platelet inhibition only, 2% were on dual antiplatelet therapy and 29% did not receive any form of anticoagulation [4]. The situation in Europe is comparible; in 2005, a Euro Heart Survey study on atrial fibrillation found oral anticoagulation to be prescribed in only 67% of patients [5]. More recently, the European PREFER in AF and the GARFIELD AF registries reported approximately 80% of hospitalized AF patients to be receiving oral anticoagulation with Vitamin-K antagonists or NOAC's [6]; However, around 20% mostly high risk (CHADs-VASc ≥3) patients still do not receive adequate stroke protection [4]; the number of patients receiving inadequate reduced dose of NOAC's is unknown.

Currently four non-Vitamin K antagonists (NOAC) are available throughout the EU. These anticoagulants, namely dabigatran, rivaroxaban, apixaban and edoxaban, have been studied in large randomized trials which also provided new insights into stroke and bleeding risk in patients with AF. Several extensive reviews are available summarizing all aspects of the different studies and specific aspects of these drugs [7, 8]. The four NOAC's compare favourably to warfarin regarding efficacy to prevent stroke and systemic embolism (Fig. 1.1) Apixaban was the only NOAC studied in comparison to aspirin (AVERROES): apixaban was clearly more effective in stroke protection and had no increased risk of bleeding in that study (Figs. 1.1, 1.2 and 1.3). Similarly, the ACTIVE-W trial found platelet inhibition to be ineffective in stroke prevention. All NOAC's reduced the number of intra-cranial bleeding significantly (Fig. 1.2), yet major bleeding using slightly different definitions in each study was similar or marginally less than with warfarin (Fig. 1.3). The benefit of reduced major bleeding is not seen in elderly patients over ≥75 years of age for the daily dosage of 2 × 110 mg dabigatran [9]. Rivaroxaban increased gastrointestinal bleeding (upper, lower, rectal) compared to warfarin (3.2% vs 2.2% overall, respectively). Recently, large registry data from health systems throughout the world with matched analysis of patients receiving Vitamin K antagonists have become available. These registries confirm the results of the randomized trials in real world scenarios for dabigatran, apixaban and rivaroxaban. The dabigatran data from the US-based Medicare system are depicted in Fig. 1.4 [10]. Similar data are available for rivaroxaban and apixaban.

The only trial comparing a NOAC to platelet inhibition is discussed here in further detail: the AVERROES trial included 5591 patients randomized 1:1 to apixaban 2 × 5 mg or aspirin (80–320 mg/day; 91% of patients received between 81 and 162 mg aspirin). Mean $CHADS_2$ score was 2.0 ± 1.1 vs 2.1 ± 1.1, respectively. 81%

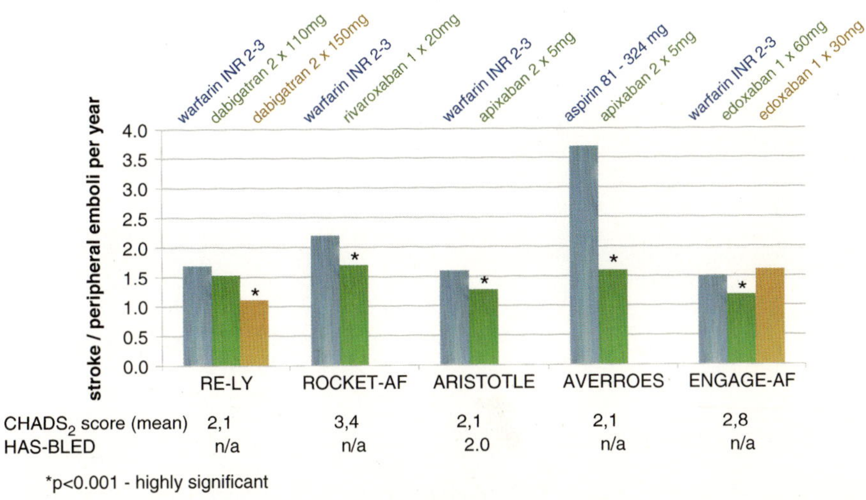

Fig. 1.1 Rate of stroke and systemic embolism in the five large studies on NOAC. Only AVERROES compared NOAC to ASS again showing platelet inhibition not to be an efficient stroke protection in patients with AF similar to earlier trials comparing warfarin and platelet inhibition like ACTIVE-W. All other studies compared NOAC to warfarin. Very similar data confirming these results are now available from large real-world registries on dabigatran, apixaban and rivaroxaban

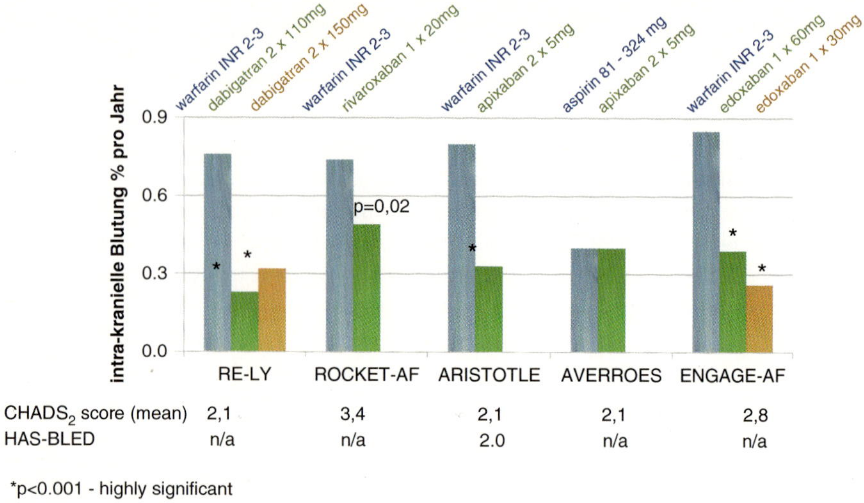

Fig. 1.2 Rate of intracranial bleeding in the five large studies on NOAC. Only AVERROES compared NOAC to ASS. Interestingly, this study finds aspirin to have the same bleeding rate as apixaban in a low-risk population. All other studies compared NOAC to warfarin

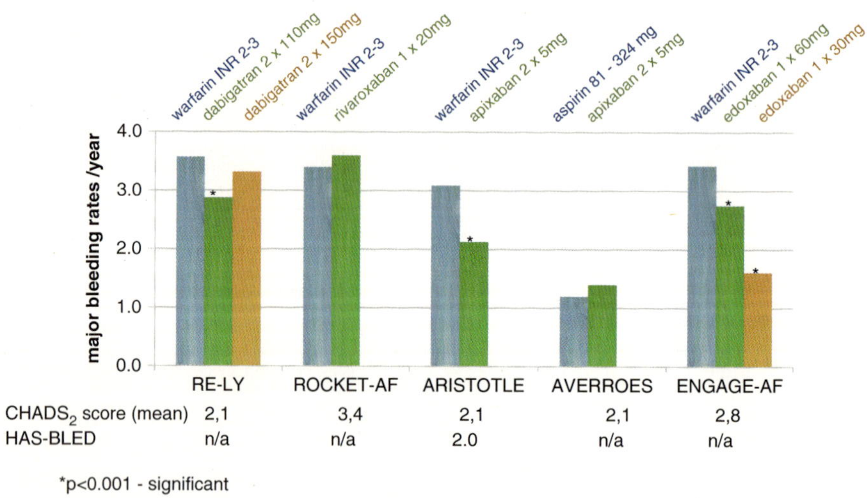

Fig. 1.3 Major bleeding rates in large NOAC trials. Patients with a history of major bleeds within a certain time frame were excluded in some trials. While rivaroxaban had no advantage over warfarin, other NOAC's had a statistically significant reduction in bleeding in this low-risk population (dabigatran 2 × 110 mg, apixaban, edoxaban). Similar data confirming these results are now available from large real-world registries on dabigatran, apixaban and rivaroxaban

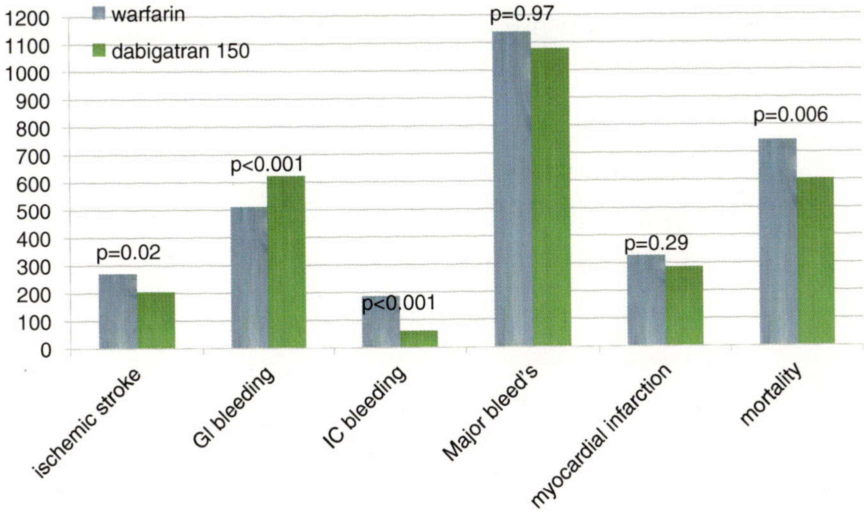

Fig. 1.4 Matched pair analysis on real-life data from the US medicare registry on dabigatran 2 × 150 mg compared to warfarin therapy in 2 × 67,202 patients. The study finds similar results to the randomized trials with less intracranial bleeding yet slightly increased gastrointestinal bleeding. The rate of ischemic stroke is significantly reduced [10]

of patients were included due to "the assessment that INR could not or was unlikely to be measured at requested intervals; uncertainty about patients ability to adhere to instructions regarding OAT, expected difficulty in contacting patient for urgent change in OAT dose or $CHADS_2$ score of one and VKA therapy not recommended by physician". A serious bleeding event in the 6 months prior to study randomization or a high risk of bleeding were key exclusion criteria. 35% of patients were recruited within Western Europe and North America, while 65% were recruited from Latin America, Eastern Europe and Asia/South Africa. As expected, apixaban reduced the number of strokes significantly compared to aspirin (1.6 vs 3.4% per year, respectively) (Fig. 1.1). Bleeding events were statistically not different between aspirin and apixaban in this trial (Figs. 1.2 and 1.3). Two different definitions were employed: while "major" bleeding occurred at a rate of 1.4 and 1.2% per year, "clinically relevant non-major" bleeding occurred at 3.1 vs. 2.7% per year, respectively. These bleeding rates as well as the low $CHADS_2$ score indicate that the study included low risk patients. The patients included in this study are therefore not representative of patients deemed to be unsuitable for oral anticoagulation in Western Europe or the US, where most patients are deemed to be ineligible for NOAC due to increased bleeding risk while INR measurements are readily available. Triple therapy combining dual antiplatelet and oral anticoagulation is a specific issue; it is now clear from various registries that there is no benefit in this treatment even regarding stent thrombosis while the bleeding risk is excessive. Combining clopidogrel and oral anticoagulation without aspirin appears to come with the lowest bleeding risk and the best outcome (Fig. 1.5).

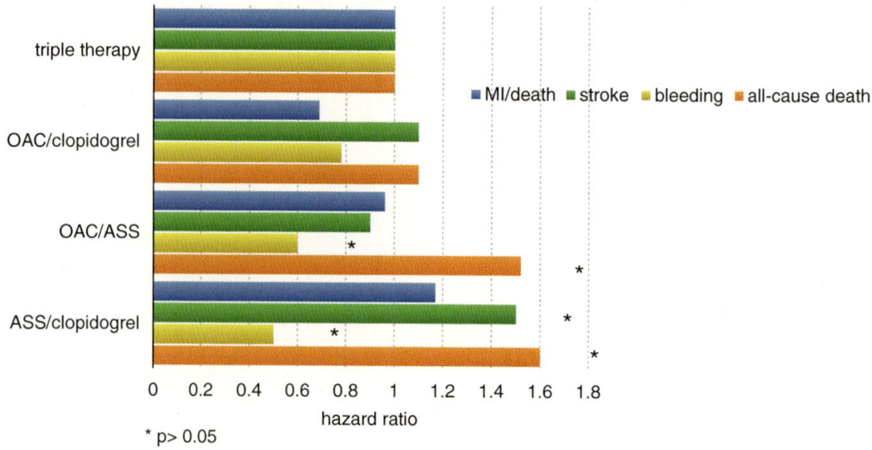

Fig. 1.5 Rate of myocardial infarction/death, stroke, bleeding and all-cause death during follow-up in 11.480 patients with atrial fibrillation and an acute coronary syndrome. Triple therapy was set at a hazard risk of one, other therapeutic options were compared. Patients on clopidogrel + OAC had the best outcome. Source: M. Lamberts et al., J Am Coll Cardiol. 2013 Sep. 10;62(11):981-9

1.4 Risk of Bleeding with Oral Anticoagulation

Many general practitioners fear the risk of bleeding and other side effects when prescribing oral anticoagulation. Several surveys indicate that prescription of oral anticoagulation is overused in younger patients with AF and severely underused in elderly patients. This is dramatic since several large studies find both the risk of stroke as well as poor clinical outcome after stroke to increase with age; this paradigm is not altered by new treatment concepts for acute stroke including thrombolysis [11]. In conclusion, stroke prevention in patients with AF is in need of new treatment options since the currently available therapies face insurmountable practical hurdles that have only partially disappeared following the introduction of NOAC's. To calculate the risk of bleeding, the 2010 ESC guidelines have introduced the HAS-BLED score based on a real-world patient cohort from the EuroHeart Survey on AF from 2005 [1]. This risk score has been derived from a patient cohort treated with warfarin. No larger studies have validated the HAS-BLED with NOAC therapy yet, however a substudy of the ARISTOTLE trial finds bleeding to increase with higher HAS-BLED score [12]. The randomized trials find extra-cranial bleeding events (i.e. gastrointestinal, bladder, skin) not to be reduced with NOAC therapy (Fig. 1.3).

Looking at NOAC prescription data in 2016 in Europe, dose reduction of NOAC therapy is performed in around 50% of patients. As the effect of NOAC's is dose dependent, dose reduction will prevent bleeding but will also reduce the effectiveness of stroke prevention. Dose reduction is clearly defined with each NOAC; in general it should be limited to patients with reduced kidney function (usually GFR < 45 ml/min), low weight (<60 kg) and/or age >80 years. Dose reduction is

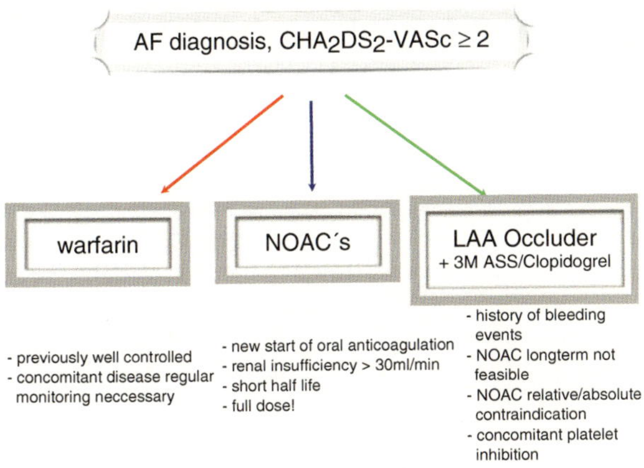

Fig. 1.6 Algorithm based on the NOAC-studies as well as the recent prospective studies on Watchman LAA occlusion. A large retrospective registry for the Amulet LAA occluder also supports this approach. LAA occluder therapy allows for stroke protection to the same degree as warfarin. Currently LAA occluder therapy is recommended for all patients that have a relative or absolute contraindication for warfarin and NOAC's at full dose. LAA occluder is followed by 3 months of dual antiplatelet therapy in most European centers

comparible to the strategy of keeping patients at an INR of 1.8 at which increased numbers of stroke do occur according to large registry data [23]. This is therefore a group of patients in which interventional stroke prevention with a LAA occluder should be performed -similar to patients with a lack of compliance or concomitant long term platelet inhibition following acute coronary syndrome events (Fig. 1.6).

1.5 Stroke Prevention in AF Patients Following Acute Coronary Syndromes

Patients with both acute coronary syndromes and atrial fibrillation are a specific group of patients with currently unclear treatment algorithms. Triple therapy (aspirin, clopidogrel, oral anticoagulation) was repeatedly shown to lead to unacceptable high bleeding rates (Fig. 1.5) also increasing clinical endpoints and mortality [13, 14]. The APPRAISE-2 study compared 2 × 5 mg apixaban on top of dual platelet inhibition after acute coronary syndrome to placebo and had to be stopped due to increased risk of bleeding including fatal and intracranial bleeding (1.3% vs. 0.5%, respectively) [15]. In contrast, the ATLAS ACS 2—TIMI 51 trial found a much lower dose of rivaroxaban (2 × 2.5 mg per day as compared to 1 × 20 mg used for stroke prevention) to be beneficial on top of dual platelet inhibition post-ACS with an acceptable increase in major bleeding (2.1 vs. 0.6% per year, respectively) but no increase in fatal bleeding [16]. Importantly, only patients with sinus rhythm were included in that trial; the low dose of rivaroxaban would not have been

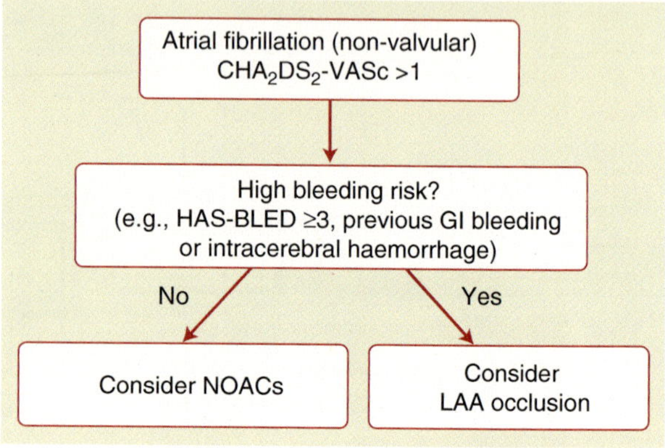

Fig. 1.7 Proposed algorithm based on a European perspective on LAA closure [22]

efficient for stroke prevention. Many centers in Europe have started to use the combination of clopidogrel and oral anticoagulation including NOAC. Several randomized trials analyzing NOAC therapy in combination with platelet inhibition are ongoing. However, the best treatment for secondary prevention of acute coronary syndromes remains the combination with new antiplatelet drugs such as prasugrel and ticagrelor. These drugs confer an even higher bleeding risk when combined with warfarin. LAA closure combined with dual antiplatelet therapy including i.e. ticagrelor or prasugrel long-term is therefore an ideal option for these patients [17] (Fig. 1.7).

1.6 Indications for LAA Occlusion in 2017

The ESC (European Society of Cardiology) guidelines on stroke prevention in AF 2016 recommend LAA occluder therapy for all patients with relative or absolute contraindication for oral anticoagulation; there is no room for platelet inhibition or reduced NOAC dose treatment (Fig. 1.8). The new oral anticoagulants show an improved efficacy and safety profile regarding stroke prevention in AF compared to warfarin. INR measurements are obsolete, which is an advantage over warfarin therapy. Due to the reduced half-life of 12 h, bridging with low-molecular weight heparin for elective surgery is not required. However,

Fig. 1.8 ESC Guidelines for stroke prevention published September 2016. (**a**) The figure summarizes stroke protection in AF: (**b**) the guideline recommendation LAA occlusion. The grading of IIbB is surprisingly unchanged in comparison to the 2012 guideline update despite a large scale of new data including prospective (EWOLUTION) and retrospective (ACP) registries as well as randomized trials (PREVAIL, 4-year PROTECT-AF data)

a

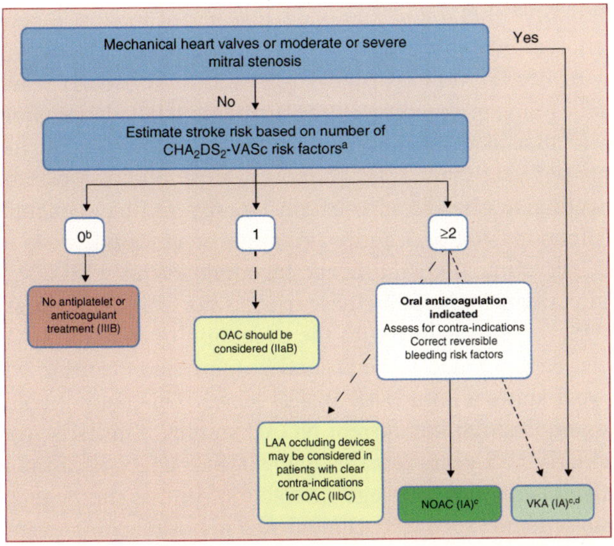

b

Recommendations for occlusion or exclusion of the left atrial appendage

Recommendations	Class[a]	Level[b]	Ref[c]
After surgical occlusion or exclusion of the LAA, it is recommended to continue anticoagulation in at-risk patients with AF for stroke prevention.	I	B	461, 462
LAA occlusion may be considered for stroke prevention in patients with AF and contra-indications for long-term anticoagulant treatment (e.g. those with a previous life-threatening bleed without a reversible cause).	IIb	B	449, 453, 454
Surgical occlusion or exclusion of the LAA may be considered for stroke prevention in patients with AF undergoing cardiac surgery.	IIb	B	463
Surgical occlusion or exclusion of the LAA may be considered for stroke prevention in patients undergoing thoracoscopic AF surgery.	IIb	B	468

AF ¼ atrial fibrillation; LAA ¼ left atrial appendage.
[a]Class of recommendation.
[b]Level of evidence.
[c]Reference(s) supporting recommendations.

patients with bleeding events and patients in need of platelet inhibition are still in need of alternative therapies. The main reason not to start a patient on oral anticoagulation remains the risk of clinically relevant bleeding which also affects quality of life; a point especially relevant to the elderly. Comparing the risk of clinically relevant bleeding in the available trials demonstrates the current dilemma in that also the new anticoagulants come with a risk of 2–3% bleeding events per year (Fig. 1.3). Moreover, most studies have only included patients that were also eligible to warfarin therapy and have excluded patients with contraindications for oral anticoagulation or at "high" risk for bleeding events, i.e. recent clinically significant bleeding events [18–20]. The HAS-BLED score of patients included in these trials is not available, yet given the fact that the $CHADS_2$ score was low with the exception of ROCKET-AF ($CHADS_2$ score 3.4) it can be estimated to be around 2. Increased bleeding with an event rate >3% per year starts with a HAS-BLED of ≥3. This patient cohort is therefore not addressed through the current NOAC studies. Similarly, optimal treatment for the elderly >75 years remains unclear. Sub-analysis of the RE-LY trial shows a significant treatment-by-age interaction, in that the benefit of the low dose dabigatran scheme (2 × 110 mg) regarding major bleeding events was eliminated in patients >75 years. More precisely, dabigatran 2 × 110 mg vs. warfarin carried a risk of 5.1% vs. 4.4% major bleeding per year in these elderly patients. Major bleeding was reported at a rate of 3.3% vs. 5.2% per year comparing apixaban and warfarin in patients aged >75 years, respectively [19].

Another group of patients in need of alternative treatment options are the patients with impaired renal function. Although both dabigatran and rivaroxaban are approved for a GFR of at least 30 ml/min at a reduced dosage, a sub-group analysis of the ROCKET-AF study observed major and clinically relevant, non-major bleeding to occur at a rate of 17.8% vs 18.3% per 100 patient-years comparing 1 × 15 mg rivaroxaban to warfarin [21]. Similar event rates are observed with apixaban and edoxaban.

The above mentioned considerations clearly demonstrate the need for interventional treatment strategies regarding stroke prevention in AF even with the new oral anticoagulants available. NOAC therapy is the standard choice for patients eligible for oral anticoagulation and who have the necessary compliance. Nonetheless, a large cohort of AF patients with a CHA_2DS_2-VASc score ≥1 not receiving OAC or in whom OAC is stopped are in need of an alternative strategy. These patients should not be treated with aspirin monotherapy, dual platelet inhibition or a reduced dose of NOAC. As summarized in Figs. 1.6 and 1.7, these patients should receive interventional LAA occlusion [22]. This approach also reflects the recently published FDA approval of the Watchman device and an expert consensus from Europe. The new AF guidelines published at the ESC annual meeting 2016 in Rome did not change the recommendation of LAA occlusion as the new data by the prospective EWOLUTION registry from Europe and the publication of the PREVAIL study both employing the Watchman device were published after the most recent guidelines had been prepared [23].

The FDA approved the Watchman LAA closure technology for patients at increased risk of stroke due to atrial fibrillation that have an appropiate reason to seek a non-drug alternative to warfarin (U.S. Food and Drug Administration, P130013). In Europe, the recently presented prospective EWOLUTION registry finds LAA occlusion with the Watchman device to be safe independent from the peri-procedural drug regimen. In fact, patients receiving NOAC therapy for the 3-months period following implantation had the lowest rates of stroke, bleeding and device-related thrombus (Bergmann et al.; EuroPCR 2016). Similar results are suggested by a large retrospective registry of the ACP device [24]. Patients were then switched to aspirin monotherapy.

LAA occlusion therapy demonstrated to be cost-effective after approximately 4 years both with the background of the US health system as well as the European perspective when compared both to NOAC therapy (high cost of drug) or warfarin (high cost for INR measurements and dose adjustments) [25–27] These data confirm LAA closure therapy to be an established part of the current treatment algorithm in patients with atrial fibrillation.

Acknowledgment The authors would like to thank Mrs. Elisa Vireca, MS, Boston Scientific, Diegem, Belgium for critical reading and helpful comments.

References

1. Camm AJ, Kirchhof P, Lip GY, et al. Guidelines for the management of atrial fibrillation: the task force for the management of atrial fibrillation of the European Society of Cardiology (ESC). Eur Heart J. 2010;31:2369–429.
2. Martinek M, Aichinger J, Nesser HJ, Ziegler PD, Purerfellner H. New insights into long-term follow-up of atrial fibrillation ablation: full disclosure by an implantable pacemaker device. J Cardiovasc Electrophysiol. 2007;18:818–23.
3. Chao TF, Lin YJ, Tsao HM, et al. CHADS(2) and CHA(2)DS(2)-VASc scores in the prediction of clinical outcomes in patients with atrial fibrillation after catheter ablation. J Am Coll Cardiol. 2011;58:2380–5.
4. Gladstone DJ, Bui E, Fang J, et al. Potentially preventable strokes in high-risk patients with atrial fibrillation who are not adequately anticoagulated. Stroke. 2009;40:235–40.
5. Nieuwlaat R, Capucci A, Camm AJ, et al. Atrial fibrillation management: a prospective survey in ESC member countries: the Euro heart survey on atrial fibrillation. Eur Heart J. 2005;26:2422–34.
6. Kirchhof P, Ammentorp B, Darius H, et al. Management of atrial fibrillation in seven European countries after the publication of the 2010 ESC guidelines on atrial fibrillation: primary results of the prevention of thromboemolic events—European registry in atrial fibrillation (PREFER in AF). Europace. 2014;16:6–14.
7. Tereshchenko LG, Henrikson CA, Cigarroa J, Steinberg JS. Comparative effectiveness of interventions for stroke prevention in atrial fibrillation: a network meta-analysis. J Am Heart Assoc. 2016;5:e003206.
8. De Caterina R, Husted S, Wallentin L, et al. New oral anticoagulants in atrial fibrillation and acute coronary syndromes: ESC working group on thrombosis-task force on anticoagulants in heart disease position paper. J Am Coll Cardiol. 2012;59:1413–25.

9. Eikelboom JW, Wallentin L, Connolly SJ, et al. Risk of bleeding with 2 doses of dabigatran compared with warfarin in older and younger patients with atrial fibrillation: an analysis of the randomized evaluation of long-term anticoagulant therapy (RE-LY) trial. Circulation. 2011;123:2363–72.
10. Graham DJ, Reichman ME, Wernecke M, et al. Cardiovascular, bleeding, and mortality risks in elderly medicare patients treated with dabigatran or warfarin for nonvalvular atrial fibrillation. Circulation. 2015;131:157–64.
11. Chandra RV, Leslie-Mazwi TM, Oh DC, et al. Elderly patients are at higher risk for poor outcomes after intra-arterial therapy. Stroke. 2012;43(9):2356–61.
12. Easton JD, Lopes RD, Bahit MC, et al. Apixaban compared with warfarin in patients with atrial fibrillation and previous stroke or transient ischaemic attack: a subgroup analysis of the ARISTOTLE trial. Lancet Neurol. 2012;11:503–11.
13. Dewilde WJ, Oirbans T, Verheugt FW, et al. Use of clopidogrel with or without aspirin in patients taking oral anticoagulant therapy and undergoing percutaneous coronary intervention: an open-label, randomised, controlled trial. Lancet. 2013;381:1107–15.
14. Lamberts M, Gislason GH, Olesen JB, et al. Oral anticoagulation and antiplatelets in atrial fibrillation patients after myocardial infarction and coronary intervention. J Am Coll Cardiol. 2013;62:981–9.
15. Alexander JH, Lopes RD, James S, et al. Apixaban with antiplatelet therapy after acute coronary syndrome. N Engl J Med. 2011;365:699–708.
16. Mega JL, Braunwald E, Wiviott SD, et al. Rivaroxaban in patients with a recent acute coronary syndrome. N Engl J Med. 2012;366:9–19.
17. Bonaca MP, Bhatt DL, Cohen M, et al. Long-term use of ticagrelor in patients with prior myocardial infarction. N Engl J Med. 2015;372:1791–800.
18. Connolly SJ, Ezekowitz MD, Yusuf S, et al. Dabigatran versus warfarin in patients with atrial fibrillation. N Engl J Med. 2009;361:1139–51.
19. Granger CB, Alexander JH, McMurray JJ, et al. Apixaban versus warfarin in patients with atrial fibrillation. N Engl J Med. 2011;365:981–92.
20. Patel MR, Mahaffey KW, Garg J, et al. Rivaroxaban versus warfarin in nonvalvular atrial fibrillation. N Engl J Med. 2011;365:883–91.
21. Fox KA, Piccini JP, Wojdyla D, et al. Prevention of stroke and systemic embolism with rivaroxaban compared with warfarin in patients with non-valvular atrial fibrillation and moderate renal impairment. Eur Heart J. 2011;32:2387–94.
22. Bergmann MW, Landmesser U. Left atrial appendage closure for stroke prevention in nonvalvular atrial fibrillation: rationale, devices in clinical development and insights into implantation techniques. EuroIntervention. 2014;10:497–504.
23. Kirchhof P, Benussi S, Kotecha D, et al. ESC guidelines for the management of atrial fibrillation developed in collaboration with EACTS: the task force for the management of atrial fibrillation of the European Society of Cardiology (ESC) developed with the special contribution of the European Heart Rhythm Association (EHRA) of the ESC endorsed by the European Stroke Organisation (ESO). Eur J Cardiothorac Surg. 2016;50(5):e1–e88.
24. Tzikas A, Shakir S, Gafoor S, et al. Left atrial appendage occlusion for stroke prevention in atrial fibrillation: multicentre experience with the AMPLATZER cardiac plug. EuroIntervention. 2015;11(10):1170–9.
25. Reddy VY, Akehurst RL, Armstrong SO, Amorosi SL, Beard SM, Holmes Jr DR. Time to cost-effectiveness following stroke reduction strategies in AF: warfarin versus NOACs versus LAA closure. J Am Coll Cardiol. 2015;66:2728–39.
26. Reddy VY, Akehurst RL, Armstrong SO, et al. Cost effectiveness of left atrial appendage closure with the Watchman device for atrial fibrillation patients with absolute contraindications to warfarin. Europace. 2016;18(7):979–86.
27. Panikker S, Lord J, Jarman JW, et al. Outcomes and costs of left atrial appendage closure from randomized controlled trial and real-world experience relative to oral anticoagulation. Eur Heart J. 2016;37(46):3470–82.

Chapter 2
Safety and Efficacy of LAA Closure

2.1 Randomized Trials on LAA Closure with the Watchman Device

As of 2017 randomized trials on LAA closure are only available regarding the single disc Watchman device. The PROTECT-AF trial compared 463 patients that were scheduled to receive LAA closure vs. 244 patients randomized to continue on warfarin [1]. The study was initiated back in 2005; participating centres had no experience with LAA closure at that time. The study aimed to show non-inferiority of LAA closure when compared with warfarin long term therapy. Close to 5000 patients with atrial fibrillation were screened in order to include a population of 700 patients into the trial (Fig. 2.1). This was due to many patients deemed to have i.e. challenging LAA anatomy difficult to occlude with the device and various other reasons (Fig. 2.1). The CAP registries and recent all-comer registries performed outside the US (see below) found successful LAA closure to be possible with the Watchman in >95% of all patients [2].

The PROTECT-AF trial included a low-risk population of patients with an average CHADs score of 2.1; V. Reddy and colleagues published the four year results in 2014. Early publications had found the initial rate of periprocedural, serious complication rate to be around 5%. In particular, pericardial effusion and periprocedural ischemic stroke emerged as an issue in these early days (Fig. 2.2). Standardization and modifications of the implantation technique have lead to a reduction of serious, non-transient complications to 0.5% even though morbidity of the patients was much higher in the recent EWOLUTION registry (CHA_2DS_2-VASc average 4.3). The non-inferiority (primary study hypothesis) of LAA closure was confirmed early on and after four years in PROTECT-AF (Fig. 2.3). Surprisingly, patients with the Watchman had an even lower cardiovascular and all-cause mortality than the warfarin group after four years [3]. The combined primary safety and efficacy endpoints (Fig. 2.4) confirmed the primary hypothesis of this trial, namely non-inferiority of Watchman LAA closure compared to

M.W. Bergmann et al., *Clinical Cases in LAA Occlusion*,
DOI 10.1007/978-3-319-51431-4_2

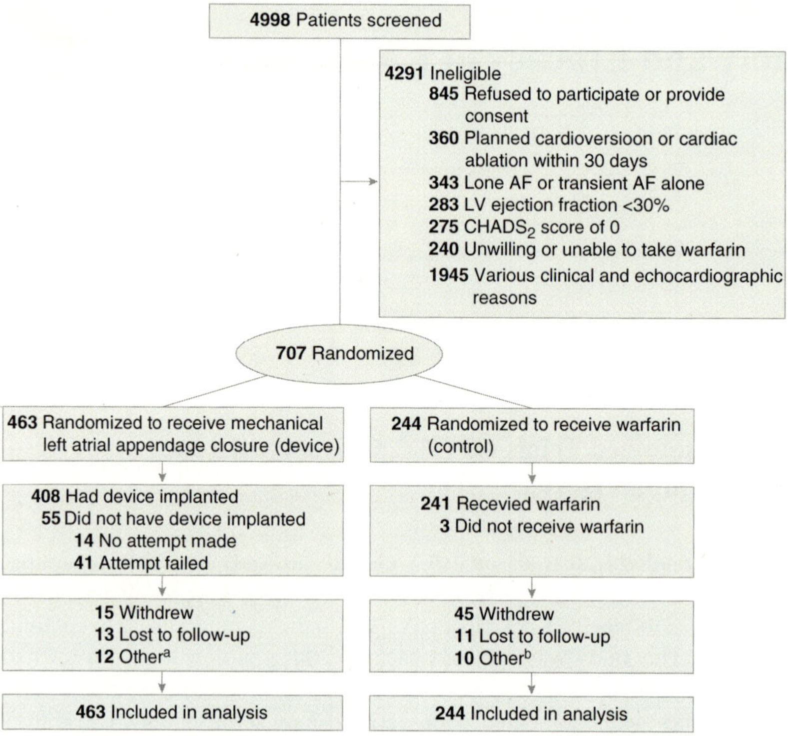

Fig. 2.1 Patient flow chart in Watchman PROTECT-AF: many patients dropped out of the study after screening due to anticipated issues with complete LAA closure in these early days of the technique [1]

	device group n=463 total events	device group events ≤ 7 days post-implant	device group events >7 days post-implant	warfarin group n=244
serious pericardial effusion	22 (4.8%)	22 (4.8%)	0	
major bleeding	22 (4.8%)	3 (0.6%)	19 (4.1%)	18 (7.4%)
procedure-related ischemic stroke	6 (1.3%)	5 (1.1%)	1 (0.2%)	
device embolization	3 (0.6%)	3 (0.6%)	0	
hemorrhagic stroke	3 (0.6%)	0	3 (0.6%)	9 (3.7%)
other	4 (0.9%)	4 (0.9%)	0	

Fig. 2.2 Primary safety endpoint of the Watchman PROTECT-AF study after 4 years of follow-up. Pericardial effusion and bleeding even under the less intense anticoagulation regime of the trial (45 days of warfarin followed by dual antiplatelet therapy until 6 months; aspirin life long) had the highest event rate in the device group while major bleeding and devastating hemorrhagic stroke occurred in the warfarin group [2, 3]

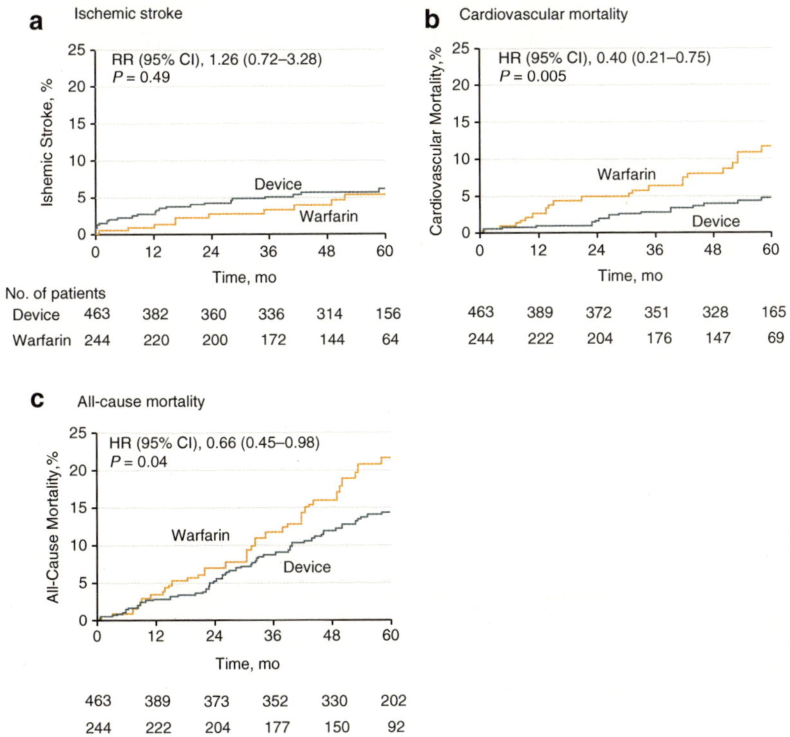

Fig. 2.3 Primary efficacy endpoints ((**a**) ischemic stroke; (**b**) cardiovascular mortality; (**c**) All-cause mortality) of the Watchman PROTECT-AF study after 4 years of follow-up. The study was designed as a non-inferiority trial; the results not only show non-inferiority but also superiority regarding all-cause and cardiovascular mortality in comparison to warfarin. The event rate of ischemic stroke was low as expected; patients in the trial had a mean CHADs score of 2.1 [3]

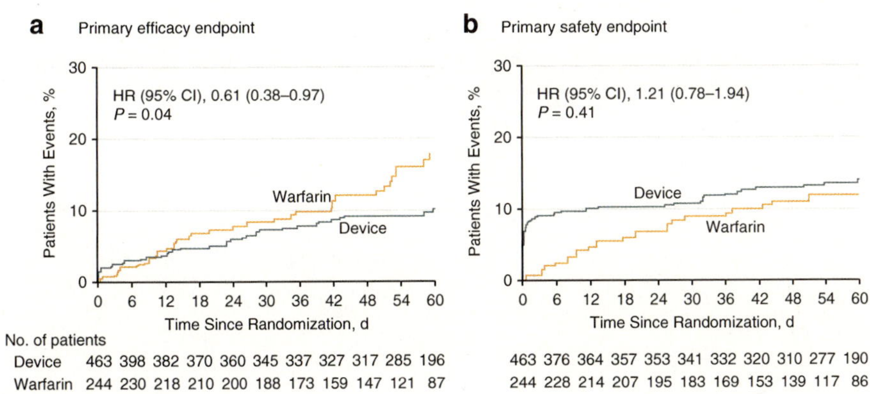

Fig. 2.4 Primary efficacy (**a**) and safety (**b**) endpoints of the Watchman PROTECT-AF study after 4 years of follow-up. Primary efficacy was defined as composite of stroke, systemic embolization and cardiovascular death. Primary safety outcome was defined as composite of major bleedings and procedure-related complications. HR indicates hazard ratio [3]

warfarin long-term treatment in patients with atrial fibrillation in need of stroke protection (CHADs ≥1). Strokes in the Watchman LAA closure group appeared to be clinically less significant than in the warfarin group with only 0.5% of disabling strokes in the device group compared to 1.2% in the warfarin group (Fig. 2.5). Interestingly, quality of life assessment in the PROTECT-AF trial showed favourable results for the device group [4]. Bleeding outcomes are also favourable for the device group [5].

The PREVAIL trial was started on request by the FDA to prove periprocedural complications to be reduced with training and the evolved implantation technique by 2009; the data provided by the PROTECT-AF and the continued access protocol registry data (CAP 1 & 2) were regarded insufficient to allow FDA approval of the Watchman device. The study included 269 patients randomized 2:1 at higher risk (mean $CHADS_2$ 2.6, see Fig. 2.6) and finished recruitment by 2012 [6]. Safety events, particular pericardial effusion, were significantly reduced to 1.7% of proce-

Event	Device Group (n = 463) Events/Patient-Years	Device Group Observed Rate[a]	Warfarin Group (n = 244) Events/Patient-Years	Warfarin Group Observed Rate[a]	Device/Warfarin Rate Ratio (95% Credible Interval)	Posterior Probabilities,% Noninferiority	Posterior Probabilities,% Superiority
Primary efficacy end point[b]	39/1720.2	2.3 (1.7–3.2)	34/900.8	3.8 (2.5–4.9)	0.60 (0.41–1.05)	>99	96
Stroke	26/1720.7	1.5 (1.0–2.2)	20/900.9	2.2 (1.3–3.1)	0.68 (0.42–1.37)	>99	83
Ischemic	24/1720.8	1.4 (0.9–2.1)	10/904.2	1.1 (0.5–1.7)	1.26 (0.72–3.28)	78	15
Hemorrhagic	3/1774.2	0.2 (0.0–0.4)	10/916.2	1.1 (0.5–1.8)	0.15 (0.03–0.49)	>99	99
Disabling[c]	8/1771.3	0.5 (0.2–0.8)	11/912.7	1.2 (0.6–1.9)	0.37 (0.15–1.00)	>99	98
Nondisabling[c]	18/1723.7	1.0 (0.7–1.7)	9/907.7	1.0 (0.4–1.7)	1.05 (0.54–2.80)	89	34
Systemic embolization	3/1773.6	0.2 (0.0–0.4)	0/919.5	0	NA		
Cardiovascular or unexplained death	17/1774.3	1.0 (0.6–1.5)	22/919.4	2.4 (1.4–3.4)	0.40 (0.23–0.82)	>99	99
Primary safety end point[d]	60/1666.2	3.6 (2.8–4.6)	27/878.2	3.1 (2.0–4.3)	1.17 (0.78–1.95)	98	20

V. Reddy et al., JAMA 2014;312 (19): 1988–98

Fig. 2.5 Intention-to-Treat primary efficacy and safety outcomes of the Watchman PROTECT-AF study after 4 years of follow-up. Observed event rate is calculated as 100 patient-years with a 95% credible interval. Primary safety outcome was defined as composite of major bleedings and procedure-related complications. Disabling or fatal stroke were defined as those with a modified Rankin score of 3–6. Note that the strokes observed in the LAA closure group were less harmful than in the warfarin group. HR indicates hazard ratio [3]

	PREVAIL trial
number of patients	269
age	74±7.4
male gender	67.7%
$CHADS_2$	2.6±1.0
stroke/TIA	27.5%

Fig. 2.6 Baseline patient data of the Watchman PREVAIL trial (V. Reddy, TCT 2014)

	Watchman	warfarin
number of patients	269	138
pericardial effusion	4 (1.5%)	0
combined primary efficacy endpoint	10 (3.7%)	5 (3.6%)
ischemic stroke	8 (3.0%)	0 (0%)
hemorraghic stroke	1 (0.4%)	2 (1.4%)
death	1 (0.4%)	4 (2.9%)

Fig. 2.7 Safety and efficacy of Watchman LAA closure in the PREVAIL trial. The primary study hypothesis, namely reduction of periprocedural safety events with a particular focus on pericardial effusion was met. Efficacy endpoints, particular ischemic stroke, was numerically higher in the device group yet particularly low in the warfarin group

dures; all but one of these effusions could be treated with pericardiocentesis (Fig. 2.7). One patient had to be operated but could be stabilized. During follow-up eight ischemic strokes in the Watchman group to none in the warfarin group were observed; the latter result was quite surprising and outside the expected range for this patient cohort. The trial was also not powered to observe efficacy of the procedure; furthermore strokes in the Watchman group were clinically less significant and rarely disabling. Further data with larger patient numbers are needed to clarify this point.

Following FDA approval of the Watchman occluder in spring 2015 further randomized trials are in planning as of summer 2016; particularly the ASAP-TOO study will provide further evidence regarding safety and efficacy of LAA closure with the Watchman device in patients ineligible to warfarin therapy. Patients are randomized to platelet inhibition vs. LAA closure with the Watchman device.

2.2 Prospective Registry Data on LAA Closure with the Watchman Device from the US

Following PROTECT-AF the participating centres were allowed to continue implanting Watchman devices within the continued access protocol (CAP) with further prospective data collection. The registries known as CAP 1 (2008–2010) and CAP 2 (2012–2014) included another 1150 patients (Fig. 2.8); they largely confirmed the results of PROTECT-AF regarding efficacy (Fig. 2.9). All the trials showed an effect of the procedural learning curve with periprocedural complications to be reduced to around 1%. During follow up, the rate of hemorrhagic stroke was significantly reduced in the Watchman group as was the rate of unexplained or

	PROTECT-AF	PREVAIL	CAP	CAP2	Total
Enrollment	2005-2008	2010-2012	2008-2010	2012-2014	
Enrolled	800	461	566	579	2406
Randomized	707	407	-	-	1114
Watchman: warfarin (2:1)	463:244	269:138	566	579	1877:382
mean follow-up, years	4.0	2.2	3.7	0.58	N/A
Patient years	2717	860	2022	332	5931

Fig. 2.8 Summary of currently available data on the Watchman device from the US. Combination of two randomized trials (PROTECT-AF and PREVAIL) together with the continued access protocol (CAP 1: continued access to PROTECT-AF; CAP 2: continued access to PREVAIL) following the studies [4]

	hazard ratio Watchman vs. warfarin	p-value
efficacy	0.79	0.22
all stroke or SE	1.02	0.94
ischemic stroke or SE	1.95	0.05
hemorrhagic stroke	0.22	0.004
CV/unexplained death	0.48	0.006
all-cause death	0.73	0.07
major bleed, all	1.00	0.98
major bleeding, non procedure related	0.51	0.002

Fig. 2.9 Combined analysis of the US randomized trials and registries: significant benefits of the Watchman group can be found for the endpoints ischemic stroke or systemic embolization, hemorrhagic stroke, cardiovascular or unexplained death and non-procedure related major bleeding [4]

cardiovascular mortality compared to the expected event rate [7]. Data were also analyzed for cost-effectiveness showing Watchman LAA closure to be effective after around 5 years in comparison to both warfarin including costs for monitoring and NOAC [5, 8].

2.3 Prospective Registry Data on LAA Closure with the Watchman Device from Europe

In Europe LAA closure emerged in 2009 and was already part of the ESC guidelines on atrial fibrillation of 2012 based on the PROTECT-AF data as well as the ASAP prospective registry performed by four centres in Germany between January 2009 and November 2011; patients with a relative or absolute contraindication for oral anticoagulation had a IIb evidence level B recommendation for the procedure [9]. The same recommendation is given in the new 2016 guidelines further supported by the new randomized trials and registries since the 2012 update; the guidelines ask for a randomized trial comparing LAA closure to NOAC therapy in order to give LAA closure a class I recommendation [10].

The ASAP study included patients ineligible to oral anticoagulation; different to the US studies (Fig. 2.8) patients received dual antiplatelet therapy following the procedure. The study confirmed safety and efficacy of the procedure also with the new post-procedural management. Further registries including the ALSTER LAA data from Hamburg found dual antiplatelet therapy to be similarly effective compared to warfarin regarding the prevention of device-associated thrombus on the device within the first three months [11]. The data have been summarized in a recent review; periprocedural complications continued to decline [12].

The European experience lead to the EWOLUTION registry which enrolled 1020 patients in 47 centres from Europe, Russia and the Middle East between October 2013 and May 2015 [13]. Data have been presented as a late breaking trial at the ESC annual conference in August 2015 and EuroPCR in May 2016. The registry included high-risk patients with a mean CHA_2DS_2-VASc of 4.6 ± 1.59 corresponding to a mean $CHADS_2$ score of 2.8 ± 1.31 (Fig. 2.10). More than 70% of patients were deemed contraindicated for oral anticoagulation. Following the procedure, only 15.6% of patients received warfarin, 11.1% received NOAC therapy and 59.6% of patients received dual antiplatelet therapy immediately after the procedure (Fig. 2.11). Severe, non-transient periprocedural complications dropped to 0.4% of patients; bleeding not associated to the procedure but the drug treatment within the first three months was the most relevant serious adverse event (Fig. 2.12). While post-procedural dual antiplatelet therapy proved to be safe and effective regarding the rate of thrombus at the device and stroke during the first three months, NOAC therapy during this time frame had the overall lowest event rate not explained by these patients to have a low risk score (Fig. 2.13).

In summary, the available prospective data on the Watchman device provide solid evidence for LAA closure to be part of the routine treatment in patients with atrial fibrillation requiring stroke prevention. In the European setting, LAA closure is cost-effective after around 4.5 years [14].

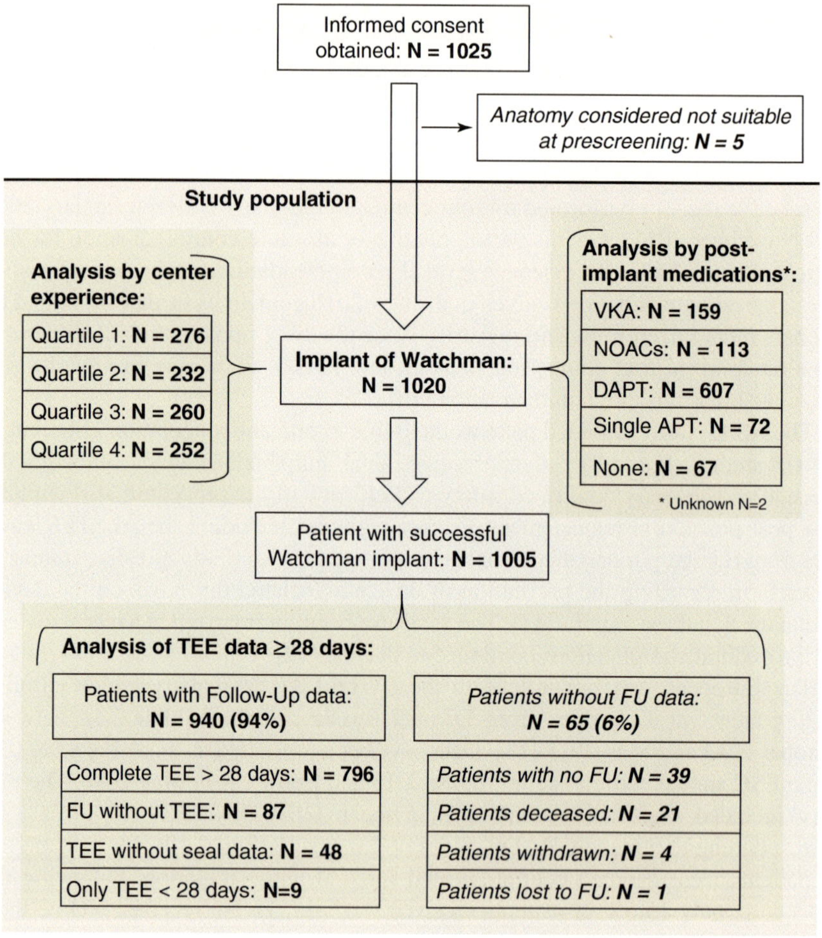

Fig. 2.10 EWOLUTION Watchman study flow chart. EWOLUTION is a prospective, 1000-patient registry with external monitoring. The all-comer study was performed in 47 sites across Europe, Russia and the Middle East. Patient recruitment started in October 2013 and finished ahead of time in May 2015. LBT EuroPCR 2016, Presenter: M.W. Bergmann

	pre-procedural	post-procedural
Nothing	27.5	6.6
Single APT	22.1	7.1
Dual APT	20.3	59.6
NOAC	14.6	11.1
Warfarin	15.5	15.6

Fig. 2.11 EWOLUTION Watchman study peri-procedural drug regimen; most patients were contraindicated for oral anticoagulation. Dual antiplatelet therapy was used in 60% of patients following Watchman implantation. LBT EuroPCR 2016, Presenter: M.W. Bergmann

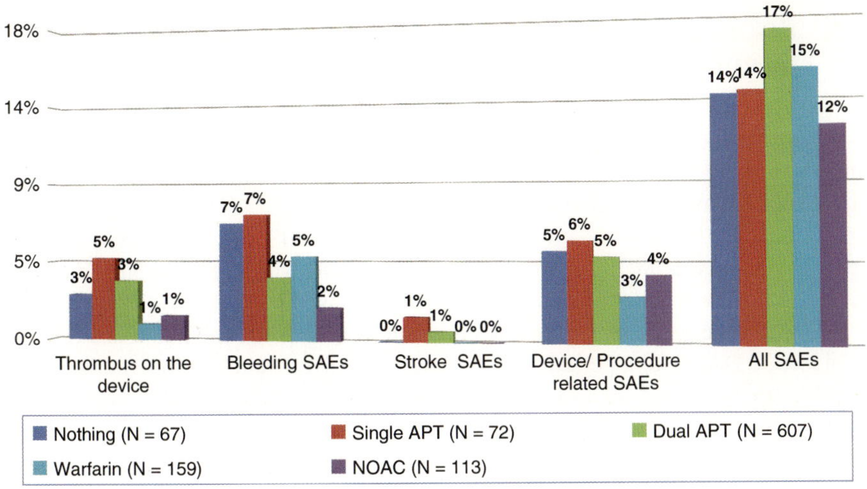

Fig. 2.12 EWOLUTION study on Watchman closure: safety events up to 92 days post-procedural stratified for post-procedural drug regimen. All drug regimen's appear to be feasible; the lowest event rate is observed with NOAC therapy post-procedural. DAPT used in the vast majority of patients in this registry has no increased risk of thrombus on the device or stroke yet comes also with a 4% bleeding risk during this time frame. LBT EuroPCR 2016, Presenter: M.W. Bergmann

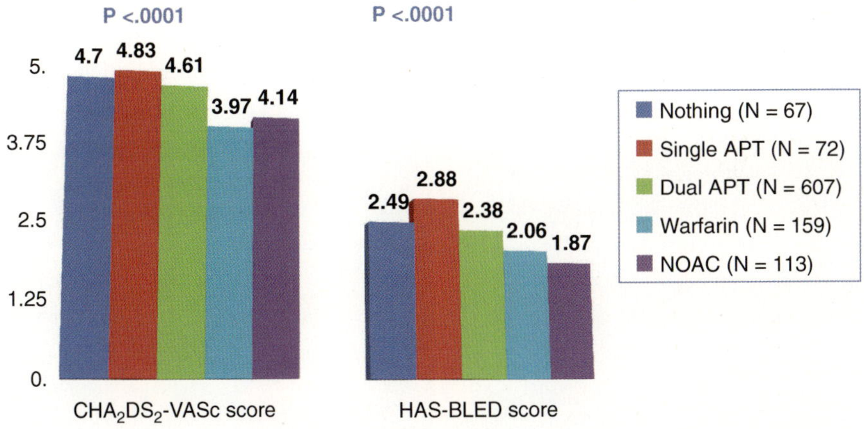

Fig. 2.13 EWOLUTION study on Watchman closure: mean stroke and bleeding risk of the various subgroups stratified for post-procedural drug regimen. Patients on platelet inhibition had a significantly higher risk of bleeding and stroke compared to the patients on oral anticoagulation in part due to higher baseline risk. Post-procedural NOAC therapy may evolve as another option. LBT EuroPCR 2016, Presenter: M.W. Bergmann

2.4 Registry Data on LAA Closure with the ACP and Amulet from Europe

The Amplatzer Cardiac Plug (ACP) multicentre registry included 1047 patients, who underwent LAA closure with the Amplatzer Cardiac Plug in 22 centres in Europe and Canada between December 2008 and November 2013. Data were retrospectively collected from each centre [15]. In this "real-world", all-comers analysis, procedural success was 98.2% and major complication rate was 5%. The main indication for LAA closure was high bleeding risk (47%) followed by previous major bleeding (35%). After the procedure, the recommendation from the device manufacturer was to prescribe DAPT for a period of 1–6 months. The average follow-up of this cohort was 13 months. Based on the estimated stroke rate per CHA_2DS_2-VASc score, there was a 59% reduction in annual stroke at follow-up (2.3% vs 5.62%). Moreover, based on the estimated bleeding rate per HAS-BLED score, there was a 61% reduction in annual major bleeding at follow-up (2.08% vs 5.34%; Fig. 2.14). The registry also found long-term stroke protection when performing a subgroup analysis of patients with >1 year follow up on aspirin or no antiplatelet or anticoagulation therapy. At TCT 2016 3 months data from a new, prospective, multicenter 1000 patient registry on the Amulet were presented as a late breaking trial by David Hiddick-Smith; the data showed comparable results to the Watchman data at that time point.

Based on the ACP Registry a number of sub-studies were performed. Kefer et al. investigated the "Impact of chronic kidney disease on LAA occlusion for stroke prevention in patients with AF" [16]. In patients with chronic kidney disease, LAA closure using the ACP had a similar procedural safety compared to patients with

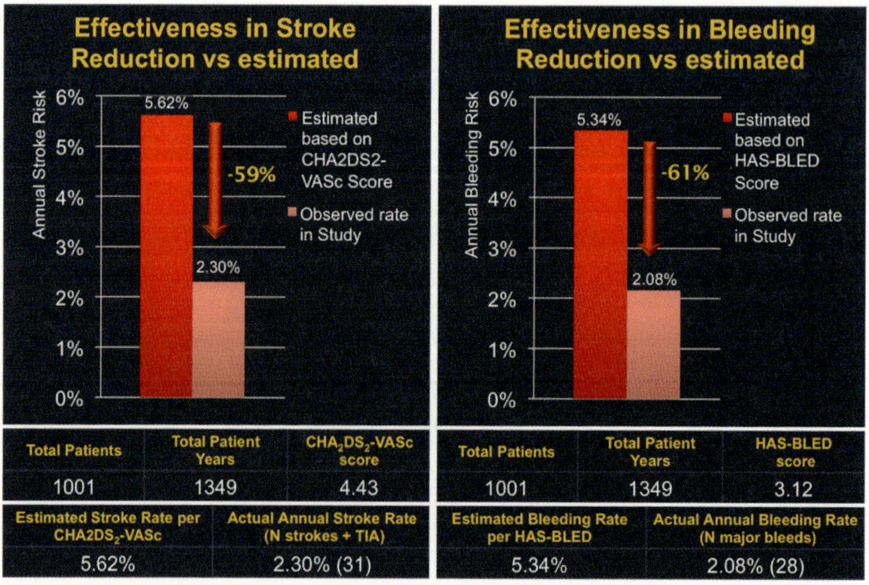

Fig. 2.14 Effectiveness of LAA closure employing the ACP LAA occluder in a large, retrospective European registry comparing estimated and observed stroke and bleeding risk. Tzikas et al., EuroIntervention 2016;11:1170–79

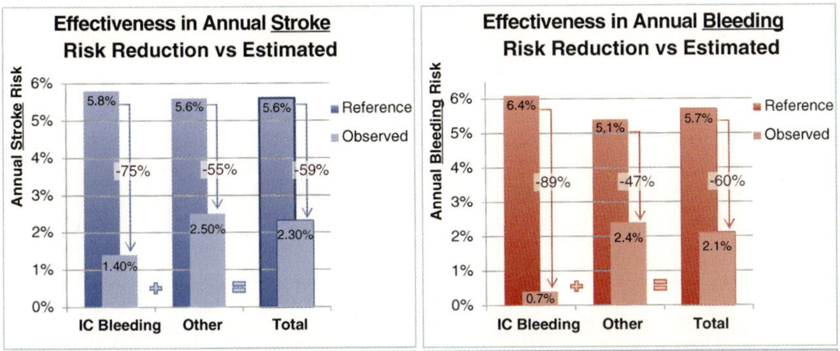

	Patients	Total Patient Years	CHA2DS2-VASc Score
IC Bleeding	188	287	4.5
Other	813	1062	4.4
Total	1001	1349	4.4

	Patients	Total Patient Years	HAS-BLED Score
IC Bleeding	188	287	3.5
Other	813	1062	3.1
Total	1001	1349	3.1

	Estimated Annual Stroke Rate per CHA2DS2-VASc	Observed Annual Stroke Rate (N strokes + TIA)
IC Bleeding	5.8%	1.4% (4)
Other	5.6%	2.5% (27)
Total	5.6%	2.3% (31)

	Estimated Annual Bleeding Rate per HAS-BLED	Observed Annual Bleeding Rate (N Bleedings)
IC Bleeding	6.4%	0.7% (2)
Other	5.1%	2.4% (26)
Total	5.7%	2.1% (28)

Fig. 2.15 Long term effectiveness of LAA closure employing the ACP LAA occluder in annual and bleeding risk. Results stratified for intracranial bleeding (IC bleeding), other events and total events. A. Tzikas et al., EuroIntervention 2016;11:1170–79

normal renal function. LAA closure offered a dramatic reduction of stroke, TIA and bleeding rate that was persistent in all stages of kidney disease. In another study, Freixa et al. explored the safety and efficacy of LAA closure in elderly (>75 years old) patients [17]. The authors concluded that LAAO was associated with similar procedural success in patients aged <75 and ≥75 years although older patients had a higher incidence of cardiac tamponade. At follow-up, stroke and major bleeding rates were similar among groups (Fig. 2.15).

The introduction of the Amplatzer Amulet for LAA closure was expected to increase procedural safety and improve clinical outcomes. In a small study by Abualsaud et al., the Amulet showed similar procedural and short-term clinical outcomes compared with the ACP [18]. However, the Amulet was associated with a significant reduction of residual leaks at follow-up. A randomized IDE clinical trial comparing LAA closure with Amplatzer Amulet versus Watchman was recently initiated in the US (first patient was enrolled in August 2016). This trial will be closely monitored by the US FDA and is expected to enrol more than 1000 patients and provide useful data on the safety and efficacy of this device compared to the Watchman device.

Acknowledgment The authors would like to thank Mrs. Elisa Vireca, MS, Boston Scientific, Diegem, Belgium for critical reading and helpful comments.

References

1. Holmes DR, Reddy VY, Turi ZG, et al. Percutaneous closure of the left atrial appendage versus warfarin therapy for prevention of stroke in patients with atrial fibrillation: a randomised non-inferiority trial. Lancet. 2009;374(9689):534–42.

2. Reddy VY, Holmes D, Doshi SK, Neuzil P, Kar S. Safety of percutaneous left atrial appendage closure: results from the Watchman left atrial appendage system for embolic protection in patients with AF (PROTECT AF) clinical trial and the continued access registry. Circulation. 2011;123(4):417–24.
3. Reddy VY, Sievert H, Halperin J, et al. Percutaneous left atrial appendage closure vs warfarin for atrial fibrillation: a randomized clinical trial. JAMA. 2014;312(19):1988–98.
4. Alli O, Doshi S, Kar S, et al. Quality of life assessment in the randomized PROTECT AF (percutaneous closure of the left atrial appendage versus warfarin therapy for prevention of stroke in patients with atrial fibrillation) trial of patients at risk for stroke with nonvalvular atrial fibrillation. J Am Coll Cardiol. 2013;61(17):1790–8.
5. Reddy VY, Akehurst RL, Armstrong SO, Amorosi SL, Beard SM, Holmes Jr DR. Time to cost-effectiveness following stroke reduction strategies in AF: warfarin versus NOACs versus LAA closure. J Am Coll Cardiol. 2015;66(24):2728–39.
6. Holmes Jr DR, Kar S, Price MJ, et al. Prospective randomized evaluation of the Watchman left atrial appendage closure device in patients with atrial fibrillation versus long-term warfarin therapy: the PREVAIL trial. J Am Coll Cardiol. 2014;64(1):1–12.
7. Gangireddy SR, Halperin JL, Fuster V, Reddy VY. Percutaneous left atrial appendage closure for stroke prevention in patients with atrial fibrillation: an assessment of net clinical benefit. Eur Heart J. 2012;33(21):2700–8.
8. Reddy VY, Akehurst RL, Armstrong SO, et al. Cost effectiveness of left atrial appendage closure with the Watchman device for atrial fibrillation patients with absolute contraindications to warfarin. Europace. 2016;18(7):979–86.
9. Reddy VY, Mobius-Winkler S, Miller MA, et al. Left atrial appendage closure with the Watchman device in patients with a contraindication for oral anticoagulation: the ASAP study (ASA plavix feasibility study with Watchman left atrial appendage closure technology). J Am Coll Cardiol. 2013;61(25):2551–6.
10. Kirchhof P, Benussi S, Kotecha D, et al. 2016 ESC guidelines for the management of atrial fibrillation developed in collaboration with EACTS: the task force for the management of atrial fibrillation of the European Society of Cardiology (ESC) developed with the special contribution of the European Heart Rhythm Association (EHRA) of the ESC endorsed by the European Stroke Organisation (ESO). Eur J Cardiothorac Surg. 2016;50(5):e1–e88.
11. Meincke F, Schmidt-Salzmann M, Kreidel F, Kuck KH, Bergmann MW. New technical and anticoagulation aspects for left atrial appendage closure using the WATCHMAN(R) device in patients not taking warfarin. EuroIntervention. 2013;9(4):463–8.
12. Bergmann MW, Landmesser U. Left atrial appendage closure for stroke prevention in non-valvular atrial fibrillation: rationale, devices in clinical development and insights into implantation techniques. EuroIntervention. 2014;10(4):497–504.
13. Boersma LV, Schmidt B, Betts TR, et al. Implant success and safety of left atrial appendage closure with the WATCHMAN device: peri-procedural outcomes from the EWOLUTION registry. Eur Heart J. 2016;37(31):2465–74.
14. Panikker S, Lord J, Jarman JW, et al. Outcomes and costs of left atrial appendage closure from randomized controlled trial and real-world experience relative to oral anticoagulation. Eur Heart J. 2016;37(46):3470–82.
15. Tzikas A, Gafoor S, Meerkin D, et al. Left atrial appendage occlusion with the AMPLATZER Amulet device: an expert consensus step-by-step approach. EuroIntervention : journal of EuroPCR in collaboration with the working group on interventional cardiology of the European society of cardiology. 2016;11(13):1512–21.
16. Kefer J, Tzikas A, Freixa X, et al. Impact of chronic kidney disease on left atrial appendage occlusion for stroke prevention in patients with atrial fibrillation. Int J Cardiol. 2016;207:335–40.
17. Freixa X, Gafoor S, Regueiro A, et al. Comparison of Efficacy and Safety of Left Atrial Appendage Occlusion in Patients Aged <75 to >/= 75 Years. Am J Cardiol. 2016;117(1): 84–90.
18. Abualsaud A, Freixa X, Tzikas A, et al. Side-by-side comparison of LAA occlusion performance with the Amplatzer Cardiac Plug and Amplatzer Amulet. J Invasive Cardiol. 2016; 28(1):34–8.

Chapter 3
Anatomy and Imaging of the LAA

3.1 Important Anatomical and Histological Aspects with Regard to LAA Closure

3.1.1 Overview

The left atrial appendage is characteristically a slender finger-like extension from the atrial body although it can also be stump-like, invoking descriptions of chicken wing, windsock, cauliflower, or cactus morphology on CT or MRI imaging. Although such graphic terms can be helpful, it is worth noting that the morphology can change, depending on the perspective and imaging plane from which the appendage is viewed (Fig. 3.1) [1].

Generally, the appendage is a flattened projection from between the anterior and lateral aspects of the left atrial chamber. Importantly, there are considerable variations in size, shape, and relationship with adjacent cardiac and extra-cardiac structures that can affect efficacy and safety of interventional procedures. The appendage tip is directed antero-superiorly with its floor (lower surface) usually overlapping the left border of the right ventricular outflow tract or the pulmonary trunk and the main stem of the left coronary or the circumflex artery (Figs. 3.1 and 3.2). In some hearts its tip is directed backwards with its body folding back upon itself while in a few hearts the tip portion passes rightward behind the arterial pedicle to sit in the transverse pericardial sinus (Fig. 3.2). The epicardial surface on heart specimens shows crenellations, or lobes. Owing to its tubular shape, its junction with the left atrium is narrow, often defined by a waist, corresponding to the ostium (or orifice) on the endocardial surface (Fig. 3.1). The position of the ostium varies, as does the length of the appendage (Fig. 3.2).

M.W. Bergmann et al., *Clinical Cases in LAA Occlusion*,
DOI 10.1007/978-3-319-51431-4_3

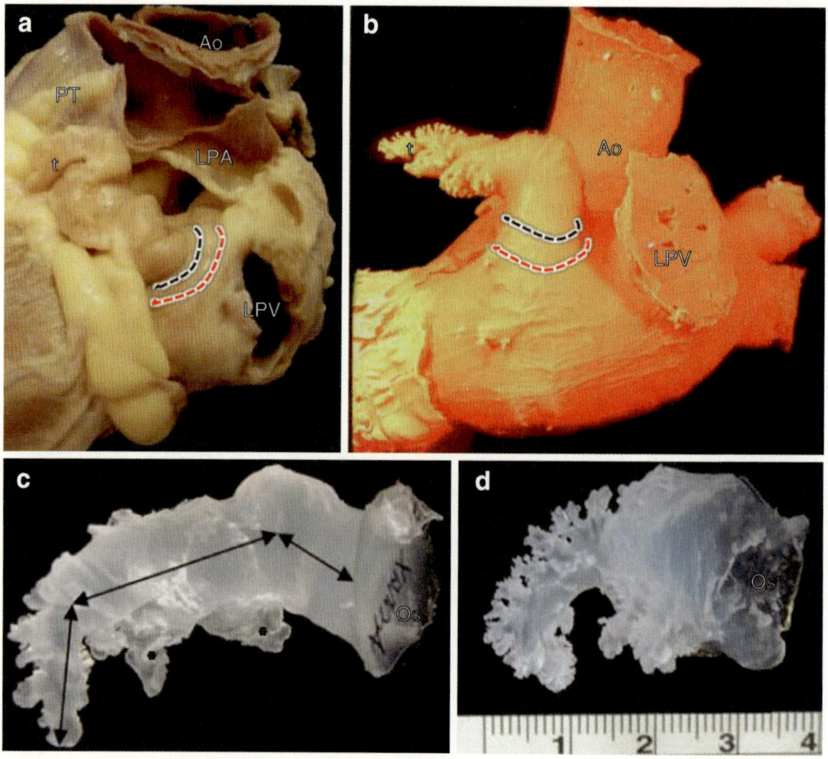

Fig. 3.1 (**a**) Shows the epicardial aspect of a heart specimen while (**b**) shows the endocast from a similar heart with common left pulmonary vein (LPV). Both are viewed from left lateral perspective to show the appendage pointing antero-cepahalad. The *red broken line* marks the ostium and the *black broken line* marks the distal margin of the neck. (**c**, **d**) are two different views of the same endocast of a left atrial appendage to demonstrate the changes in morphology. *Double arrows* mark the bends and the asterisks indicate the lobes. Ao = aorta; LPA = left pulmonary artery, Os = ostium, PT = pulmonary trunk; t = tail of appendage

3.1.2 Important Surrounding Structures

The fibrous pericardium surrounds the heart. Relevant to manoeuvres in the pericardial space to reach the appendage is the course of the left phrenic nerve which descends on the fibrous pericardium in the vicinity of the roof of the appendage [1, 2]. A study on cadavers revealed that the course of the left phrenic nerve and its accompanying pericardiophrenic vessels in the fibrous pericardium was overlying the tip of the appendage in 59% and over the neck of the appendage in 23% [2].

The major branches of the left coronary artery also run on the epicardial surface and overlap the appendage to a varying extent. Furthermore, on the epicardial aspect the left coronary lymphatic channel formed from the union of the anterior interventricular trunk and the obtuse marginal trunk passes beneath the left atrial appendage

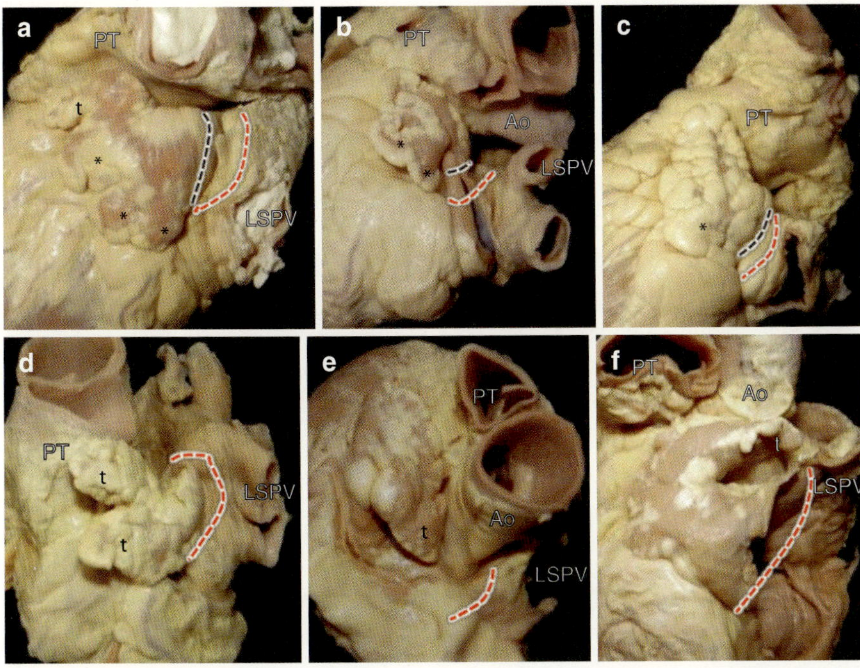

Fig. 3.2 Approximately left lateral perspectives of the left atrial appendage to show the variability in morphology, lobes (*), location of the ostium (*red broken line*), and length of the appendage's neck (*black broken line* denotes distal margin). (**a**, **b**) have anteriorly directed ostium related to the orifice of the left superior pulmonary vein (LSPV) whereas (**c**) has a laterally directed ostium. The lower three panels show variations in the tip(t) portion of the appendage. (**d**) A bifid appendage. (**e**) The appendage body is folded over. (**d**) the tip is in the transverse sinus behind the aorta. Abbreviations as in Fig. 3.1

close to the ostium. The anterior interventricular cardiac vein on its ascent continuing as the great cardiac vein that runs into the atrioventricular groove also passes underneath the appendage but its course tends to veer away from the ostium.

3.1.3 The Left Atrial Appendage

The juncture of the appendage with the atrial body is the ostium (or orifice) so the appendage is deemed to be the structure extending from the ostium to the tip. Veinot and colleagues [3] described a lobulated body portion and a tail portion. The lobes are defined as protrusions from the appendage body whereas the tail portion may bend but not produce new lobes at the point of flexion (Fig. 3.2). Eighty percent of the 500 heart they examined had two lobes or more. Although the appendage has a general flattened shape, the lobes and tail are not all aligned on the same plane (Fig. 3.2).

3.1.3.1 Ostium

When viewed from inside the left atrium, the ostium leading to the appendage is not perfectly round (Fig. 3.3). Instead, it is commonly oval in shape or tear-drop shaped with mean long diameter of 17.4 ± 4 mm and short diameter of 10.9 ± 4.2 mm as measured on postmortem hearts [1]. On the endocardial surface, the superior and posterior borders of the ostium are well demarcated by the left lateral ridge

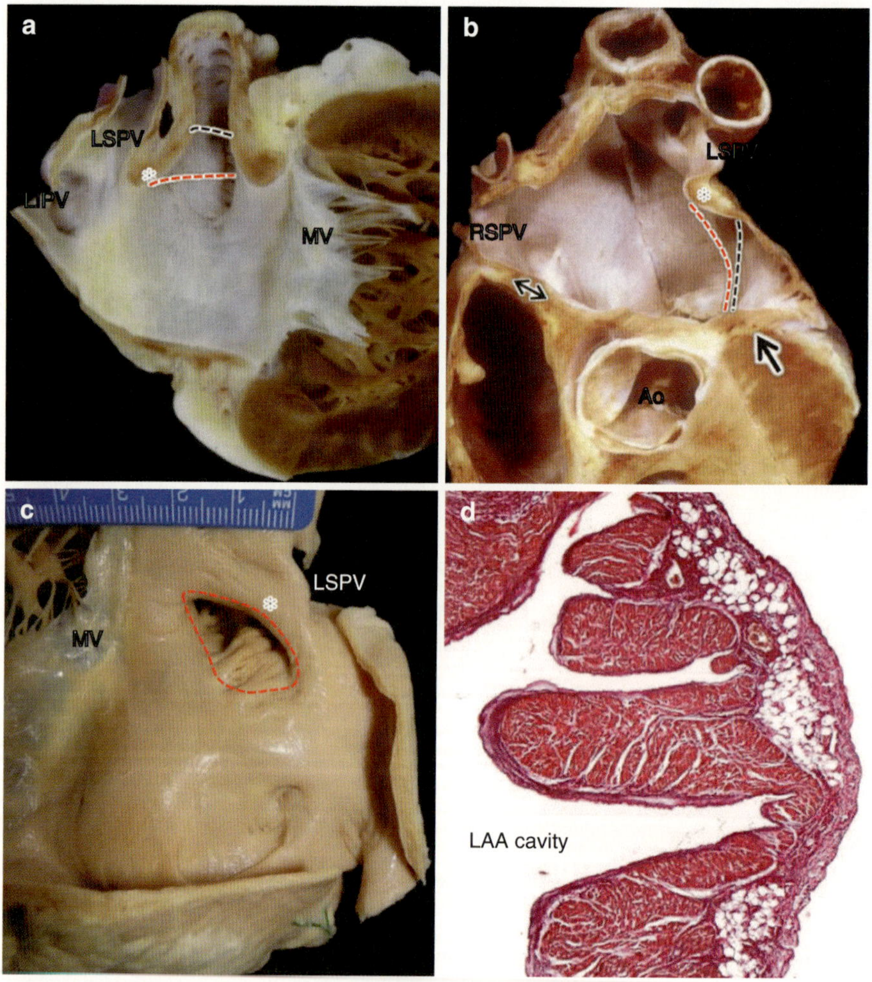

Fig. 3.3 (**a**, **b**) simulate TEE long axis and short axis cuts respectively to show the relationship between the left lateral ridge(*) and the left pulmonary vein orifice. The proximal (*red broken line*) and distal margin of the neck (*black broken line*) are indicated. The *arrow* in (**b**) points to the circumflex artery. The *double arrows* mark the plane of the atrial septum. Note the proximity of the aortic root to the anterior margin of the septum. (**c**) Shows endocardial aspect of the ostium. Proximal to the ostium the free left atrial wall without any trabeculae or pectinated muscles is visible. The ridge between the superior and posterior borders marks the ostium (*red broken line*). The muscle bundles distal to the ostium located within the appendage are clearly visible. (**d**) A histologic section through the appendage wall shows the paper-thin area in between the muscle bundles prone to perforation

separating it from the orifices of the left pulmonary veins. Lacking a ridge, the anterior and inferior borders are less well-defined. Nevertheless, there is a perceptible narrowing of the left atrium in this region. Notably, the smooth atrial wall is often punctuated by pits and troughs in this pre-ostium region. The floor of these indentations is extremely thin, comprising of little more than a few myocytes sandwiched between epicardium and endocardium [1].

Commonly known as Coumadin ridge, the left lateral ridge is actually an infolding of the left atrial wall which contains within it the vein or ligament of Marshall and also a left atrial artery that occasionally supplies the sinus node of the heart (Fig. 3.3). This so-called ridge varies in extent, size and in cross-sectional profile. In cases with narrow ridges, there is increased risk of dual-disk device implants obstructing drainage of the adjacent pulmonary vein. From heart to heart, the ostium of the appendage varies in its relationship with the pulmonary venous orifices. Most common is the ostium situated in an antero-superior position relative to the left superior pulmonary vein. Least common is the location of the ostium antero-inferior to the left inferior pulmonary vein orifice whereby the distance between the anterior and inferior margins of the ostium to the mitral annulus is reduced [4].

3.1.3.2 Neck

There is usually a tubular portion of the appendage leading from the ostium to the wider lobulated body. This neck region varies in length and in morphology (Fig. 3.2). Those with short necks, with or without an early lobe close to the ostium, or has sharp angulation of the appendage body, may not be suitable for implanting devices that plug into the appendage. In hearts with a funnel shaped neck, its distal margin may be interpreted as the appendage ostium instead [4]. On imaging, however, the ostium is sometimes taken at the level of Coumadin ridge whereas the neck (and the landing zone) is deeper into the appendage at the level of the circumflex artery (Fig. 3.3).

3.1.3.3 Appendage Body

The body is lobulated (Fig. 3.2). Its cavity is lined by a complex arrangement of muscle bundles of varied thicknesses interspersed with paper thin atrial wall in between (Fig. 3.3). At the interface between upper and lower walls the bundles may be strut-like with variations of thin bundles and thicker branching bundles. On imaging, some thicker bundles appearing like thrombi or intraatrial masses need careful evaluation.

3.1.4 The Atrial Septum

Crossing the atrial septum to reach the ostium of the appendage requires understanding of the septal components. The thin flap valve of the oval foramen that is fused to the muscular rim of the foramen represents the site of the true atrial septum.

This area is better seen on the right atrial side as a depression surrounded by a slightly raised rim in many cases although the distinction between the two structures are not clear in approximately 18% of individuals [5]. The rim is a muscular filled with fibro-fatty tissues of the epicardium and termed the interatrial groove (or septal raphe). Crossing though the thicker tissues of the fold may result in a less maneuverable catheter than crossing through the thin flap valve. Care should be taken not to exit the heart into the transverse pericardial sinus or into the aortic root when crossing anteriorly outside the rim. The variable locations of the ostium (Fig. 3.2) may require careful assessment of the optimal position for puncture in order to reach the target site.

3.2 Pre-Procedural Imaging of the LAA

As the broad variety in LAA anatomy impacts device selection, implantation strategies and procedural efficacy an accurate assessment of anatomic LAA characteristics is mandatory before a LAA occlusion procedure. The orifice of the LAA is typically located laterally and superiorly with the LAA body typically extended between the anterior and lateral walls of the left atrium (LA) and the tip directed antero-superiorly. There are substantial variations in LAA anatomy to consider that impact device selection and procedural success. The LAA ostium is generally oval in shape with diameters ranging from 10–40 mm [1, 3]. A very eccentric LAA ostium implanted with a round-shaped device may have an increased risk of peri-device leakage. In comparison with normal sinus rhythm, atrial fibrillation (AF) is associated with larger LAA volumes by up to three times normal size [6], therefore patients with chronic AF will most likely need larger device sizes.

Determining the depth and orientation of the main anchoring lobe is also an important aspect for LAA occlusion procedures. The number and origin of additional LAA lobes also influences implantation strategy. More than 50% of patients have two or more lobes [3]. If a lobe originates very close to the LAA ostium it may remain unsealed after device placement. When there are two large lobes with a bifurcation close to the ostium or a chicken wing morphology is present specific implantation strategies are often needed.

Imaging modalities used to evaluate the LAA routinely include transthoracic (TTE) and transesophageal echocardiography (TEE) and occasionally multidetector computed tomography (MDCT) or magnetic resonance imaging (MRI).

3.2.1 Transthoracic Echocardiography

Two-dimensional (2D) and three-dimensional (3D) TTE are not adequate to characterize the LAA anatomy, but they are useful prior to a planned procedure to assess LA dimensions, volumes and function. In addition, left ventricular (LV) function has to be evaluated, as it is an important factor for stratifying the risk for thromboembolism as determined by the CHA_2DS_2-VASC score [7]. Contraindications for LAA closure that can also be identified by TTE include rheumatic mitral valve (MV) disease resulting in valvular AF, the presence of thrombi in the cavities of the LA or LV or pericardial effusion that is more than small in size. Patients with severe mitral stenosis or other valvular diseases requiring surgical repair or patients with mechanical heart valves who require chronic anticoagulation therapy should not be considered for LAA closure procedures.

3.2.2 Transesophageal Echocardiography

As the LAA morphology cannot be definitely assessed by TTE a TEE is essential and is considered as the main imaging modality in the pre-procedural evaluation of the LAA. In the majority of patients the close anatomical relationship of the LA and the esophagus results in excellent imaging quality and allows for a detailed LAA assessment [8].

First, a thrombus in the LA or LAA has to be excluded by TEE [9, 10]. In most cases 2D TEE, which has a higher spatial resolution compared to 3D, is sufficient to exclude a thrombus, but in some cases 3D TEE may be helpful in differentiating a thrombus from a large pectinate muscle [11]. Figure 3.4 shows an example of a 2D TEE view and an enface 3D view of the LAA that verifies the presence of a prominent tissue bridge formed by pectinate muscles, thus allowing the exclusion of a thrombus.

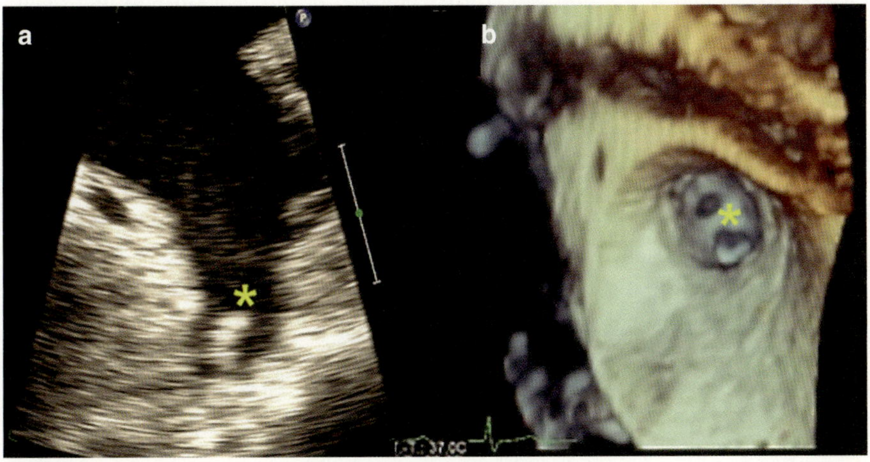

Fig. 3.4 *Differentiation of a thrombus from pectinate muscles in the LAA by 3D TEE*. In (**a**) a 2D TEE 90° view shows an echodense structure in the distal part of the LAA (marked with a *yellow star*). The corresponding 3D TEE enface view (**b**) clarifies, that this structure is a pectinate muscle bridge. A thrombus could therefore be excluded

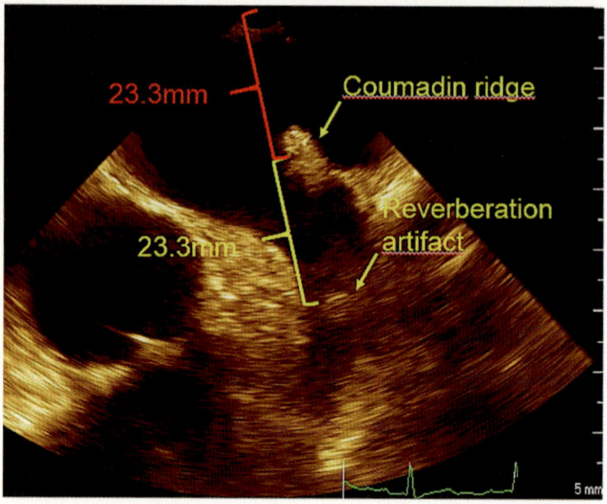

Fig. 3.5 *Left atrial appendage artifact (reverberation) seen inside the LAA*. No clear attachment to the LAA wall of the reverberation artifact can be observed. The measurements (*red and yellow brackets*) show, that the artifact is twice the distance from the transducer as the Coumadin ridge. Note, the prominent Coumadin ridge itself may be misdiagnosed as a thrombus in this patient. The lack of mobility and the typical location helps to distinguish it from a thrombus

Reverberation artifacts have also been described in the LAA. It could be demonstrated that 23% of patients had structures in their LAA which were interpreted as artifacts [12]. All artifacts were located twice the distance from the transducer as from the Coumadin ridge. The position and echogenicity markedly differs from LAA thrombi. Unlike the artifacts, all thrombi found in the LAA were attached to the LAA wall and had a uniform consistency and different texture to that of the LAA wall. None of the artifacts were attached to the LAA wall and the consistency was not uniform (Fig. 3.5). A prominent Coumadin ridge (ligament of Marshall) can also be misdiagnosed as thrombus. The lack of mobility and the typical location, most commonly best seen in a mid-esophageal two-chamber view, usually helps to distinguish it from an abnormal structure as seen in Fig. 3.5.

As demonstrated in Fig. 3.6, the use of color flow Doppler with a reduced pulse repetition frequency (PRF) or an ultrasound contrast agent may also be helpful in determining the presence of a thrombus. Tissue Doppler has also been used to distinguish true thrombus from pectinated muscle or tissue: thrombus appears with altered movement from the surrounding tissue when analyzed image by image.

If a thrombus in the LA or LAA is verified, the procedure should be postponed in order to avoid iatrogenic thromboembolism caused by clot dislodgement by a catheter or a device during device placement. In the presence of a LA or LAA clot anticoagulation therapy should be given until the thrombus has resolved as determined by repeat TEE imaging (a TEE is usually repeated after 4-6 weeks). If a thrombus persists, case reports have been presented that describe safe LAA occlusion by using carotid protection devices like the Claret device (Sentinel).

Other potential sources of systemic embolism such as cardiac masses and aortic arch atheroma also need to be excluded. 3D TEE is a very useful adjunct to conventional

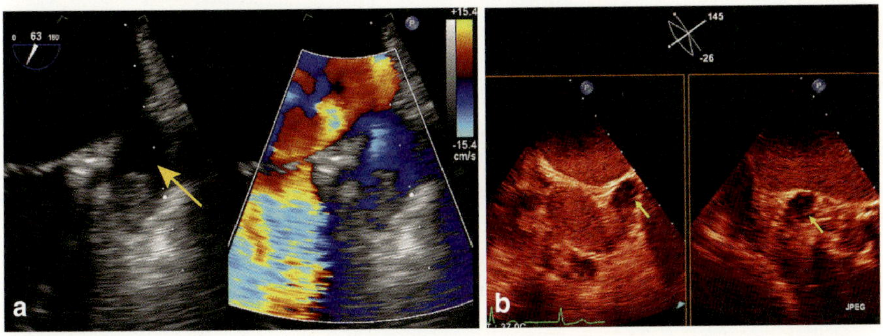

Fig. 3.6 (**a**, **b**) *Imaging with color flow Doppler and ultrasound contrast agent for thrombus detection*. In (**a**) a thrombus (*yellow arrow*) within the LAA cavity is seen (*left*) that is spared out in color Doppler imaging with a reduced pulse repetition frequency (PRF = 15.4 cm/s) (*right*). (**b**) gives an example of a thrombus (*yellow arrow*) in the very distal part of a chicken wing morphology that is spared out from ultrasound contrast in X-plane imaging

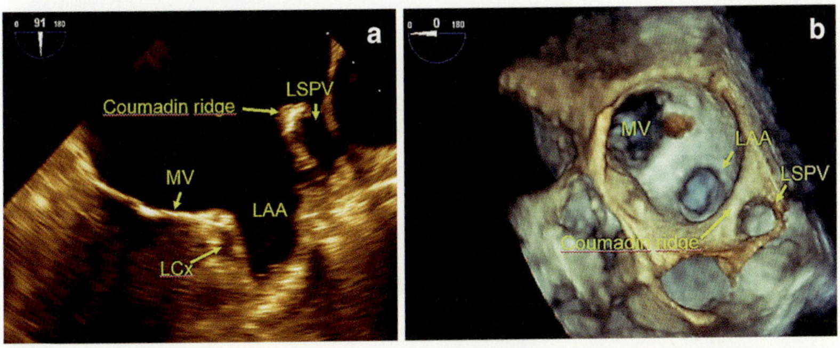

Fig. 3.7 (**a**, **b**) *Neighboring structures*. The relationship of the LAA to neighboring structures is shown in a 90° 2D TEE (a) and a 3D wide angle enface view from the left atrium (**b**). LCx = left circumflex coronary artery; MV = mitral valve; LAA = left atrial appendage; LSPV = left superior pulmonary vein

2D imaging as it renders more accurate information on surface features, diameters, volumes, mobility, spatial relationship to neighboring structures and exact location and origination of such intracardiac masses [13–16].

A systemic infection as well as an active endocarditis constitutes a contraindication for LAA closure and must be ruled out by laboratory parameters and TEE imaging [17].

As transseptal puncture (TSP) is most commonly used to place the catheter and LAA occlusion device into the LAA, careful evaluation of the interatrial septum in regard to mobility, thickness, the presence of an interatrial septum aneurysm, atrial septal defect(s) (ASD) or a patent foramen ovale (PFO) is necessary. The left superior pulmonary vein (LSPV) should be assessed for obstruction and the mitral valve for any kind of pathology. Figure 3.7 shows that these two structures are adjacent to and located in close proximity to the LAA ostium and have a low but potential risk of interference with a LAA occlusion device.

3.2.2.1 Anatomical Imaging of the LAA

In order to understand the complex 3D morphology of the LAA a careful multiplane 2D TEE analysis should be performed. Scanning through the LAA by rotating the TEE probe from 0° to 180° [18] with the probe position in the high or mid-esophageal region is recommended. It is important to define the number as well as the exact origination of additional lobes and identify and characterize all lobes accurately.

The depth of the LAA is evaluated by angiography (preferably by using an atraumatic pigtail catheter) and by TEE imaging. The view that shows the maximal depth of the LAA is typically optimal for the evaluation of the long axis of the LAA. It is usually found in a short axis TEE plane between 45° and 70°. The left circumflex coronary artery (LCx) can be identified in this view at the medial side of the LAA and the limbus (also known as Coumadin ridge) to the left superior pulmonary vein which defines the lateral border of the LAA (Fig. 3.8). These structures play a role

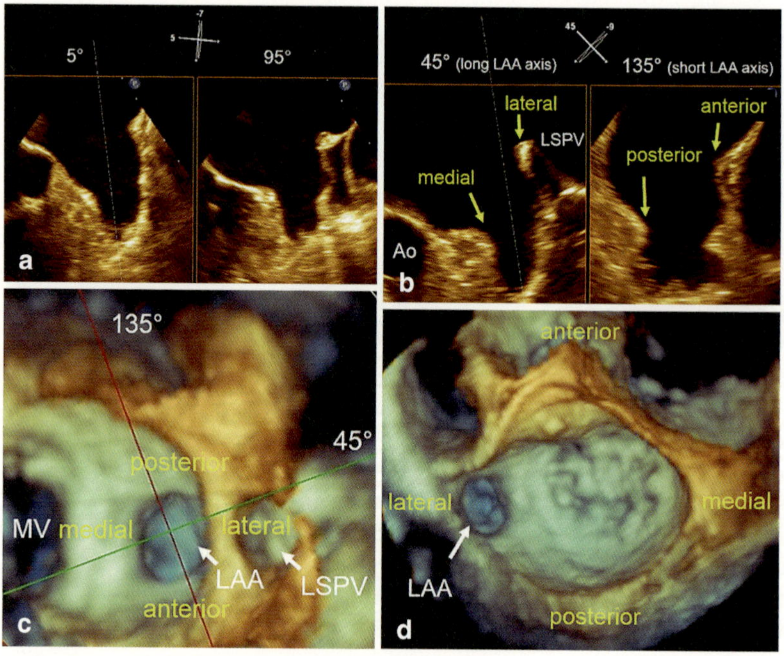

Fig. 3.8 (**a–d**)*Anatomical imaging of the LAA*. The recommended views for LAA evaluation (~0°,~45,° - 90°, ~135°) are easiest obtained by using X-plane imaging as demonstrated in (**a**, **b**). The 45° view and the 135° view allow for an evaluation of the LAA borders in an anatomical orientation (**b**). In (**c**) a 3D enface view demonstrates the axis of the 45° plane (*green line*—defines the lateral and medial border of the LAA) and the axis of the 135° plane (*red line*—defines the anterior and posterior border of the LAA) in the same patient. The longest depth can be observed in the 45° view (**b**) thus indicating a more lateral than anterior position of the LAA ostium which is confirmed in a 3D enface view from the LA (**d**). (**e**) *Example of a left atrial appendage that originates anteriorly*. The maximum length of this LAA is measured in a 10° view with the aorta in the view thus indicating that this LAA ostium is originating more anteriorly. This is confirmed in a 3D TEE enface view (bottom right). Ao = aorta; MV = mitral valve; LAA = left atrial appendage; LSPV = left superior pulmonary vein

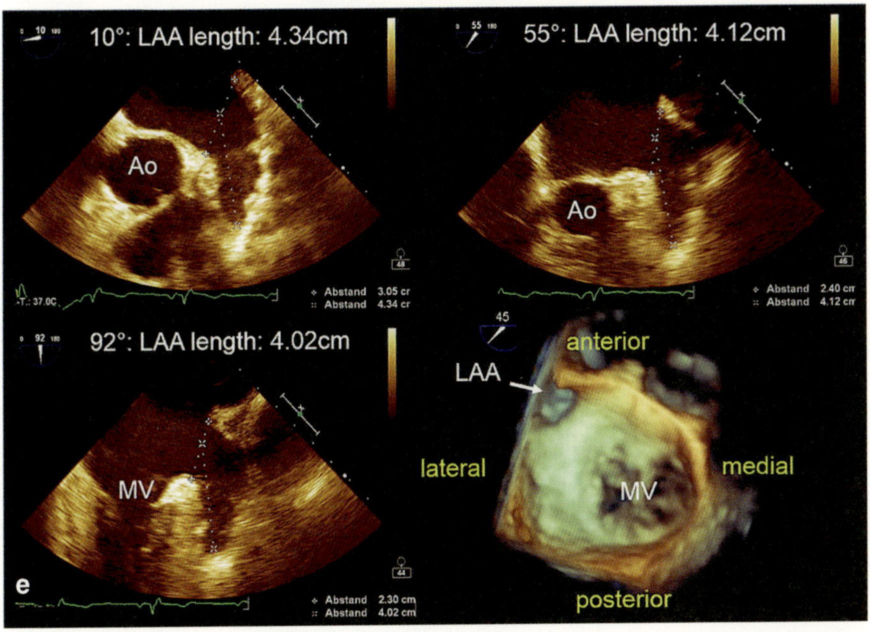

Fig. 3.8 (continued)

as important landmarks for the sizing process as described later. In cases where the LAA originates more anteriorly, the longest depth is usually seen in an image plane <45° and the aorta will be visible in the view. In cases where the LAA originates more laterally the long axis and consecutively the longest depth of the LAA can be appreciated best in planes >60° (up to 90°). In these imaging planes the aorta is not in the imaging plane (and thus is not seen), but the MV comes into the view. The origination and the course of the LAA in antero-lateral orientation should be evaluated as it has impact on the choice of the TSP site and the selection of an appropriate curve of the delivery sheath as illustrated in Fig. 3.9. With 3D TEE imaging this information can be obtained in a single wide-angle enface view that includes the MV (positioned in the middle of the image), the interatrial septum on the medial side and the LAA on the lateral side of the MV as demonstrated in Fig. 3.8.

The short axis of the LAA can be readily assessed using X-plane imaging (an imaging modality that comes with 3D imaging). When a 45° view optimally shows the long axis of the LAA a corresponding orthogonal 90° view is automatically rendered by the system and a 135° (45° + 90° = 135°) (Fig. 3.8) imaging plane of the short axis of the LAA is shown. The cropping of a 3D data set also can render these views. When X-plane imaging is not available the 135° view can also be achieved by conventional 2D imaging. To get optimal image quality it is thereby sometimes necessary to slightly pull back the TEE probe to position it slightly higher in the esophagus.

The 135° imaging plane is particularly important. First, larger ostium diameters can more frequently be found on imaging planes showing the short axis of the LAA between 120° to 135° rather than at 45° or 90° [19] due to the elliptical shape of the

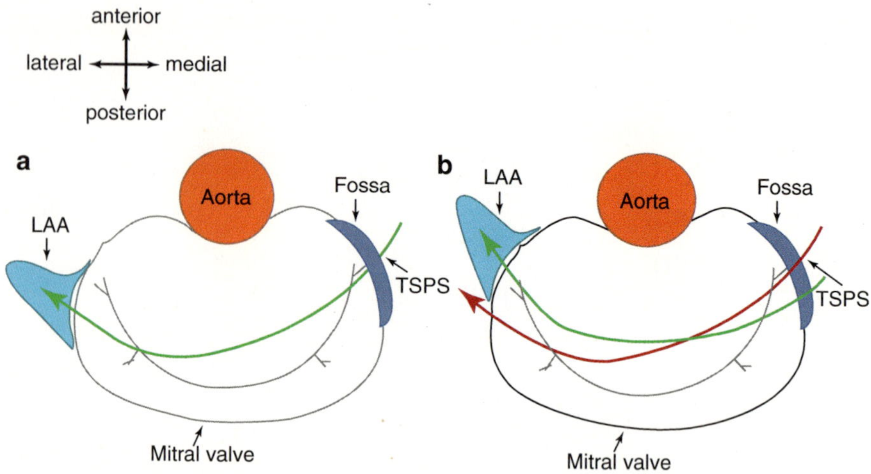

Fig. 3.9 Schematic to illustrate the impact of the location of the LAA orifice on the transseptal puncture site (TSPS). In (**a**) the LAA is located more laterally. The chosen TSPS in the mid-fossa and the usage of a specific sheath curve (illustrated by a *green arrow*) result in a coaxial entry into the LAA. In (**b**) the LAA is located more anteriorly and the usage of the same TSPS and sheath curve does not allow for a coaxial entry into the LAA (illustrated by a *red arrow*). Coaxial entry into the LAA in this case can be achieved by choosing a more posteriorly located TSPS as illustrated with the *green arrow*. LAA = left atrial appendage; TSPS = transseptal picture site

LAA ostium in most of the cases. As the largest measurement of the ostium diameter usually dictates the size of the selected device it is crucial to obtain measurements in this view. Secondly, in this view the anterior and posterior borders of the LAA can be appreciated (Fig. 3.8). The posterior part of the LAA is of major importance as this is the region where the protrusion of the devices from the LAA into the LA is more pronounced and where peri-device leakages after device deployment most commonly occur. Therefore it is mandatory to assess this region with particular caution after device placement.

Thirdly, we have found, that a chicken wing morphology is generally best evaluated using planes between 120° and 135°. Recognizing this specific morphology adequately may have implications on implantation strategies [20, 21]. The depth of the LAA is typically shortest in this imaging plane.

LAA morphologies which make device implantation more challenging should also be carefully identified before a planned procedure because this may have impact on the device selection and/or on the implantation strategies. Table 3.1 provides an overview of potentially challenging LAA morphologies.

3.2.2.2 Device Specific Measurements

Successful percutaneous LAA closure requires careful sizing of the dimensions at the plane where the device will be seated after release. This plane is commonly referred to as the “landing zone”. Optimal matching of LAA dimensions and device size

Table 3.1 Overview of some potentially challenging LAA morphologies

Morphology	Challenges	Potential strategy
Seondary lobe originating close to the ostium	This lobe may not be covered after device placement	An Amulet device may be preferable as the proximal disc may cover the ostial area. A Watchman device should be anchored in the anterior/superior lobe with proximal expansion covering the inferior lobe
Two large lobes with a bifurcation close to the ostium	Device may be captured in one of the lobes and the other lobe stays unsealed	An Amulet device may be used when the remaining depth is ≥10 mm. Alternatively a Watchman device can be implanted off axis in an oblique position
Very short LAA	Not enough space to accomodate a device with standard implantation techniique	A Watchman device may be implanted with less depth by pushing distally after release of 50% of the device
Very large LAA landing zone	A landing zone diameter >31 mm is larger than the required diameters for a Watchman occluder or an Amulet device	Two small Watchman devices ("kissing Watchman") may be considered. A LARIAT suture system may also be an option (diameters <40 mm in CT evaluation are required)
Very small LAA landing zone	A landing zone diameter <11 mm is smaller than the required diameters for a Watchman occluder or an Amulet device	Oversizing of an Amulet occluder or a Watchman device may be accepted. A LARIAT suture system may be considered
Cone shaped LAA (high ostium/landing zone ratio)	The ostium diameters are considerably larger than the landing zone dimensions and the disc of an Amplatzer occluder may be too small for adequate sealing	A Watchman device may be preferable; if an Amulet occluder is used the device may need to be oversized to cover the ostium adequately
Chicken wing morphology	Most likely small LAA depth, short neck, early bending may occur and anchoring may be difficult	A "sandwich technique" should be considered when using an Amulet device; distal anchoring with a Watchman device is another option
Proximal LAA membranes or septae	Access to the LAA may be difficult or impossible with an endoluminal device	A LARIAT suture system may be considered

ensures a stable device position, optimal sealing of the LAA and limits reposition of the device. An undersized device carries the risk of device migration or even embolization and increase risk of peri-device leakages [20]. Conversely, extreme oversizing of the device should also be avoided because of the risk of LAA perforation which may be followed by the development of a pericardial effusion as well as cardiac tamponade [22, 23]. Precise knowledge of the dimensions of the landing zone is therefore particularly important in selecting the appropriate device size (Table 3.2).

In order to avoid undersizing all measurements of LAA dimensions should be performed at the diastole of the LA (end of ventricular systole) and normal LA

Table 3.2 Overview of applications for different imaging modalities in the assessment of the LAA

Imaging modality	Main imaging tasks	Application: Patient selection	Procedure planning	Procedural guidance	FU
2D/3D TTE	LA diameter, volume and function LV function for risk stratification (CHA_2DS_2-VASC Score) LA/LV thrombi/ intracardiac masses Evaluation of contraindications Pericardial effusion	yes	yes	no	yes
2D/3D TEE	Thrombus exclusion (LA/LAA)- (less accurate with ICE) Exclusion of other sources of embolism (e.g.cardiac masses, aortic arch atheroma) (not possible with ICE) Evaluation of contraindications Number and origin of additional lobes Localisation of the LAA orifice (more anterior or more lateral) Evaluation of neighbouring structures (LSPV/ MV) Evaluation of the interatrial septum (mobility/ thickness/aneurysm/ PFO/ASD) Measurements for device selection Evaluation of challenging LAA morphologies Monitoring and guidance of procedural steps Monitoring of complications during the procedure (Pericardial effusion, tamponade, thrombi, device migration-embolization) Assessment of the final result after device positioning (device release criteria/stability) Assessment of TSP site Follow-up evaluation (pericardial effusion, thrombus detection, peri-device leaks, stable device position)	yes	yes	Yes (ICE can be used as alternative option during the procedure)	yes
MDCT and MRI	Alternative imaging options to TEE (used for the same imaging tasks as TEE- see above)- can render additional or supplementary information Mostly used when TEE is not suitable Currently not used for procedural guidance	yes	yes	no	yes

filling conditions (LA pressure should be at least 10 mmHg; dehydration of the patients leads to incorrectly smaller measurements [24]).

During device insertion, the landing zone must be defined and measured in TEE images and with fluoroscopy according to the specific requirements of the device that is chosen. The landing zone plane is usually located slightly below the anatomical LAA ostium in the neck region of the LAA (the neck constitutes a tubular junction between the ostium and the deeper lobar region of the LAA). When 2D TEE imaging is used, measurements are most commonly obtained in at least four different high to mid-esophageal views: typically at ~0°,~45°,~90° and ~135°. As mentioned above, due to the oval shape of the LAA the largest measurements are most likely obtained in the 135° view. Several studies validated that 3D TEE measurements are closely related to CT measurements [25, 26] whereas 2D measurements tend to underestimate ostium and landing zone areas [25–28]. To obtain 3D measurements, 3D enface images for direct measurements are not recommended as the plane of the landing zone can not be well defined. 3D measurements should be obtained by using 3D cropping tools which allow the precise definition of the landing zone plane.

Device selection is usually based on the maximum diameter, yet oval shaped LAA landing zones may also lead to oversize the device in certain cases. Similar to the experience with other sizing algorithms particularly for transcatheter aortic valve replacement, the calculation of a mean LAA landing zone diameter (either by dividing the maximum diameter by the minimum diameter or by using perimeter or area rendered values) and the choice of the device size according to these values seems reasonable. However, the official sizing recommendations refer to the maximum LAA dimension for device size selection and most interventionalists follow this reference.

In addition, the depth of the LAA has to be measured in the expected axis of the selected device to ensure, that the anchoring lobe is big enough to accommodate the selected device. Measurements are usually documented in mm.

Device specific measurements for the two devices that are currently most frequently implanted (the Watchman occluder and the Amulet device) are described in detail in the text that follows below.

Five sizes are available for the Watchman LAA occlusion device: 21, 24, 27, 30 and 33. Measurements for this device are performed from the level of the LCx or alternatively the level of the MV (caudal part of the LAA) to a point 1–2 cm distal from the tip of the Coumadin ridge to the left superior pulmonary vein (cranial part of the LAA). The required landing zone diameters for the Watchman device range from 17–31 mm. The largest dimension usually dictates the device size which is typically selected 3–6 mm larger than the measured dimensions. A device compression of 15–30% should be achieved after deployment to ensure a safe engagement to the LAA wall [29]. The depth of the LAA is usually measured angiographically by markers located on the Watchman delivery sheath negotiating the depth of the LAA over a 6F pigtail catheter as a rail. Depth measurements by TEE are obtained by performing a more or less perpendicular measurement to the landing zone plane (small deviations of the angle are acceptable). As the length of the device progressively increases as device diameter increases, larger devices need larger depth dimensions (same depth as device diameter). Figure 3.10 shows an example of a TEE measurement for a Watchman device.

The Amulet device constitutes of two components: a lobe which serves as an anchoring mechanism and a disc that is responsible for the sealing of the LAA ostium. Both are connected via a flexible waist. Eight device sizes are available: 16,18, 20, 22 mm (lobe length 7.5 mm, waist length 5.5 mm, disc size = lobe size + 6 mm) and

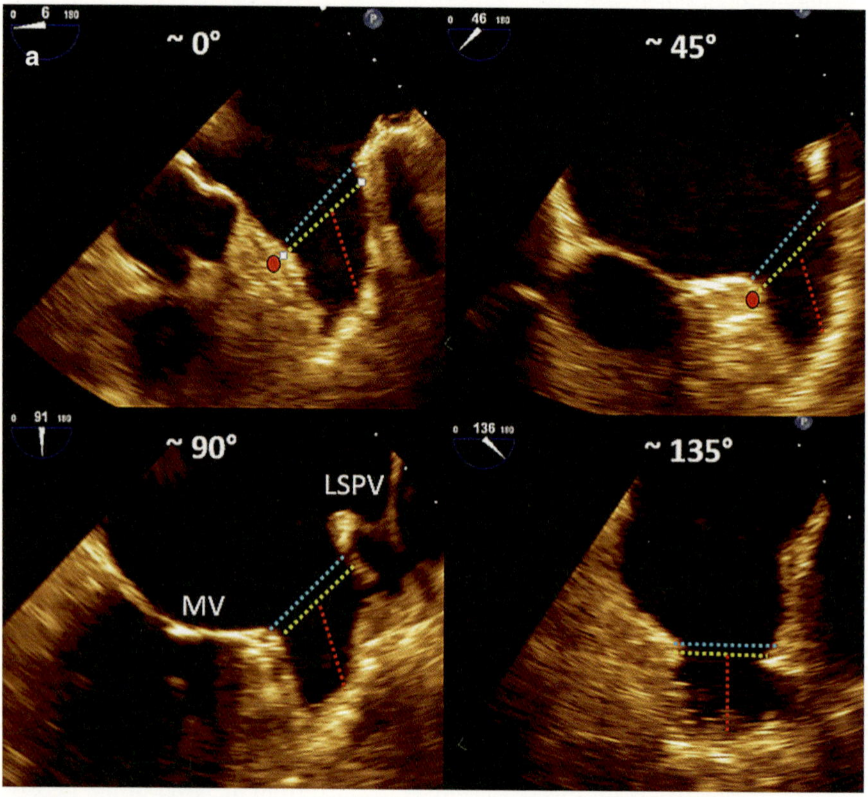

Fig. 3.10 (**a**, **b**) *Sizing for a Watchman device* (**a**) and *an Amulet occluder* (**b**): the osital plane is illustrated by a blue dashed line, the landing zone measurement by a *dashed yellow line* and the depth in the axis of the device by a *dashed red line*. As illustrated in a for a Watchman device the landing zone measurement is performed from the level of the LCx (*red dot*) or the MV to a point 1–2 cm below the tip of the Coumadin ridge. Note, the landing zone is usually located slightly below the ostial plane. The depth is measured perpendicular to the landing zone measurement. The landing zone measurement for the Amulet device is performed approximately 10–15 mm into the lobe either parallel to the ostial plane (*blue dashed line*) or, in case the Coumadin ridge is short and it is intended to cover the entire proximal area parallel to a line that is drawn to the tip of the Coumadin ridge as shown in b (*green dashes line*; upper right and lower left image). The depth is measured perpendicular to the landing zone plane.

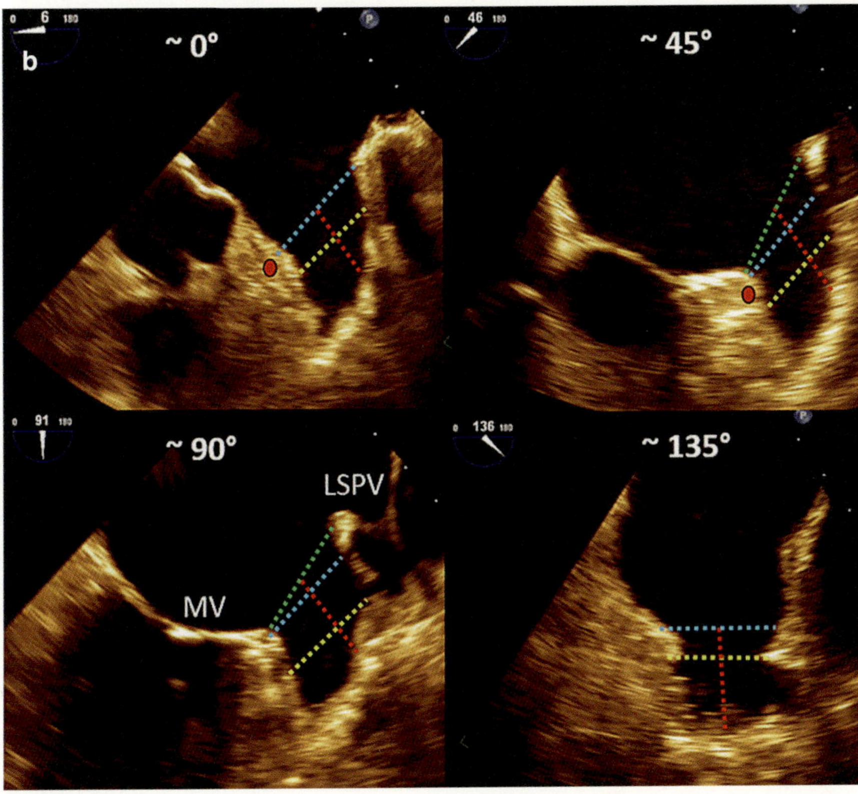

Fig. 3.10 (continued)

25, 28, 31 and 34 mm (lobe length 10 mm, waist length 8 mm, disc size = lobe size + 7 mm). Due to this device construction measurements are performed differently. The landing zone in the anchoring lobe is measured approximately 10–15 mm distal from the ostial plane into the lobe. The level of the LCx or the MV serves as a landmark. Required landing zone dimensions range from 11–31 mm. Sizing for the disc is done separately at the proximal plane of the coumadin ridge or, in case there is a relatively short Coumadin ridge a measurement to the tip of the Coumadin ridge is performed in order to try to cover the entire ostial region with the disc. It has to be ensured that the disc size of the selected device size is big enough to cover the LAA ostium. The depth has to be measured in the axis of the neck (perpendicular to the landing zone plane; small deviations of the angle are acceptable). A LAA depth of ≥12 mm is required to accommodate this device. An example of a measurement for an Amulet device is demonstrated in Fig. 3.10 (b).

In some patients more than one landing zone is conceivable. In these cases measurements should be performed for all potential landing zones.

3.2.3 Computed Tomography and Magnetic Resonance Imaging

Although TEE is most commonly used for the evaluation of the LAA, multi-detector computed tomography (MDCT) and cardiac magnetic resonance imaging (MRI) are also evolving as valuable additional technologies for pre-procedural assessment of LAA anatomy and function, the detection of LAA thrombi and the post-procedural evaluation of device position and complications [30] particularly in patients who are not suitable for TEE. Currently neither method is used in the catheterization laboratory for procedural guidance.

MDCT renders 3D volumetric data sets of the entire heart (and extra-cardiac structures if needed) with high spatial and temporal resolution. Reconstructions along different planes at different time points during the cardiac cycle allow for an adequate morphological assessment of the LAA.

While it has an excellent sensitivity for excluding thrombi in the LAA (up to 100% [31]) MDCT has a high rate of false positive results and poor intraobserver variability [32].

It has been shown, that perimeter derived measurements of the LAA ostium by CT were most reproducible for sizing and selecting an LAA occluder device rather than selecting the device according to the maximum diameter as it is currently recommended in the instruction manual for use for the Watchman as well as for the Amulet device [33, 34]. It can be expected that these MDCT findings will have an impact on sizing algorithms once they are confirmed by TEE.

MDCT was also used to classify different LAA shapes: most commonly a chicken wing morphology was found (48%), other morphologies like a cactus, windsock and cauliflower were seen in 30%, 19% and 3% respectively [35]. It was found that a chicken wing morphology was less frequently associated with a history of stroke than other LAA morphologies [35, 36]. Device implantation strategies may be influenced by these specific morphologies (examples will be given in Chap. 8 for the use of an Amulet device and in Chap. 6 for the use of a Watchman device), but the impact of these different morphologies on procedural outcome after implanting an LAA device remains unclear. In addition, with TEE imaging or contrast angiography the determination of such a morphology can be challenging as the same LAA may have a different appearance in different planes.

For a better pre-procedural planning, pre-acquired 3D CT data sets can be processed with dedicated software that is currently available (e.g. 3mensio Medical imaging BV, Bilthoven, Netherlands). This software provides facilitated segmentation and cropping tools, sizing algorithms and allows for an overlay of defined measurements (e.g. the landing zone) on a fluoroscopic image that is also generated. These features are helpful in selecting an appropriate device size and in depicting the best angiographic angle for device implantation (Fig. 3.11). During follow-up exploration CT may be helpful in assessing peri-device leakages [37] and intracardiac thrombi or thrombus material that is attached to the device and pericardial effusion.

The need for ionizing radiation constitutes a disadvantage and has to be taken into consideration when performing a CT. MRI is another non-invasive imaging

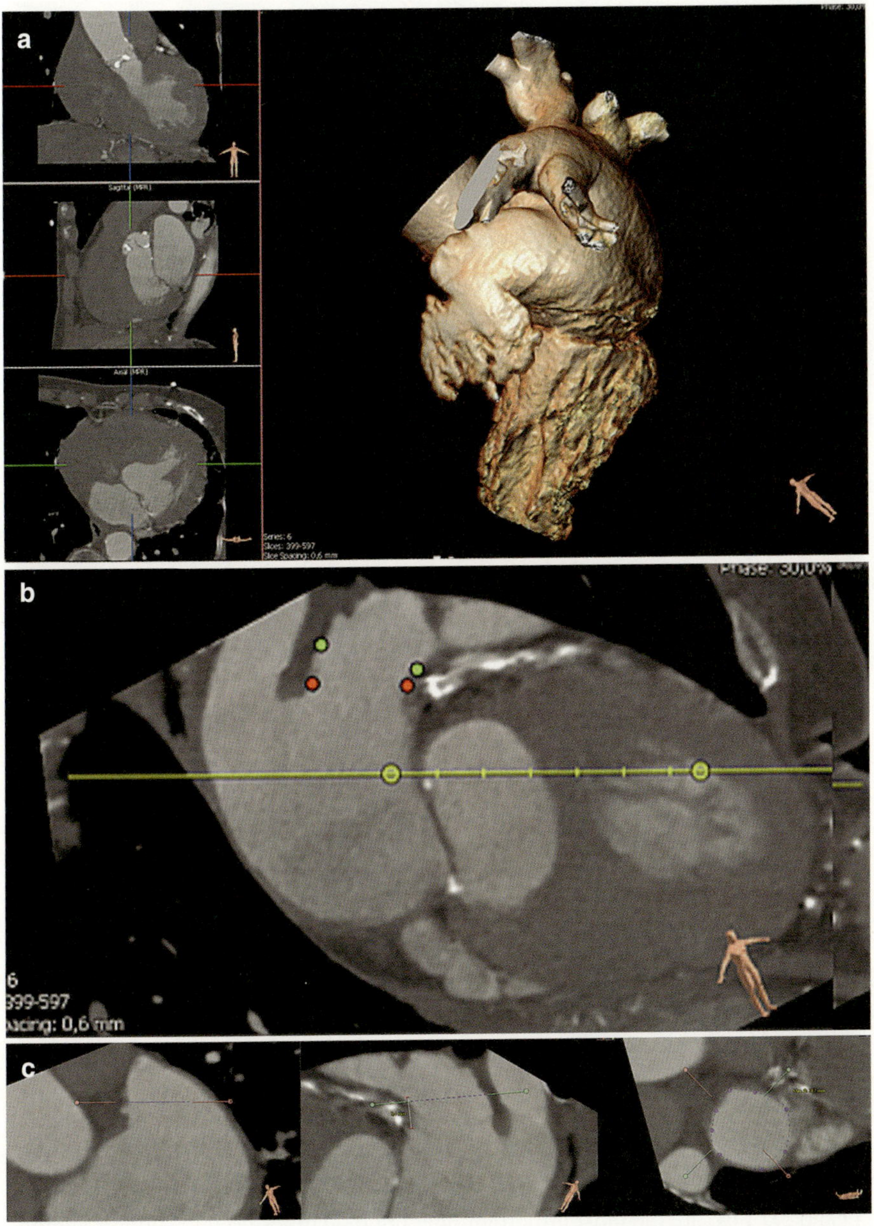

Fig. 3.11 (**a**, **b**) *Planning of a LAA closure procedure by using 3D computed tomography reconstruction software* (3mensio Medical Imaging, Bilthoven, Netherlands). (a) shows the automated segmentation of the left atrial appendage (with a chicken wing morphology in this case). The ostial plane (*red dots*) and the landing zone plane (*green dots*) are then defined by placing markers as seen in (**b**). (**c**) In the next step measurements of the ostium (not shown) and the landing zone (shown in this image) are performed in different planes. Diameters (*left* and *middle*) can be measured as well as areas and perimeters (*right*). (**d**, **e**) The defined ostial plane (*orange circle*) and the landing zone (*light green circle*) are seen in CT images (**d**) and can be overlayed on a generated fluoroscopic image (**e**). This allows for the determination of the best fluoroscopic angle for device implantation

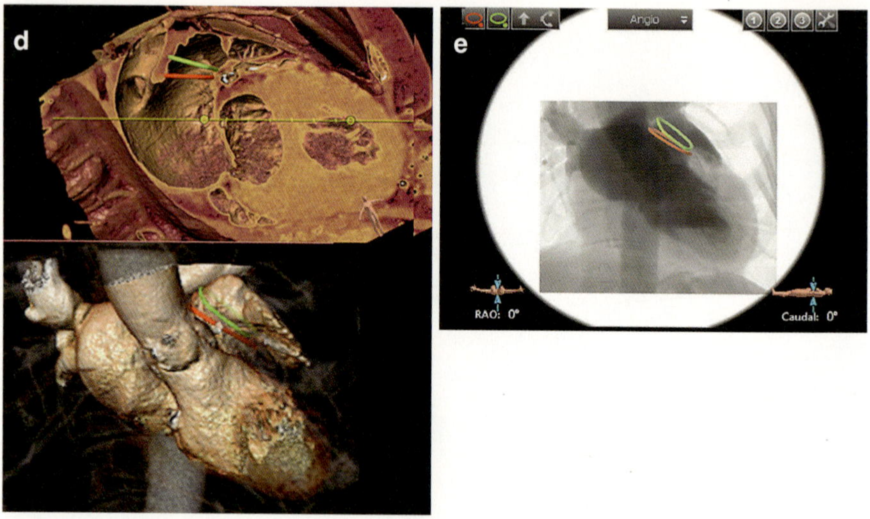

Fig. 3.11 (continued)

option in pre- and post-procedural evaluation of the LAA although there is less experience with this modality than with CT. Assessment of the LA and LAA sizes and function as well the exclusion of a thrombus in patients with AF can be performed with similar accuracy compared to TEE [38–41]. After device deployment contrast-enhanced MRI can be used to assess device position and to detect residual flow from the LA into the LAA cavity [42]. It is safe to image the Watchman device with MRI. It has been clinically evaluated and tested and findings show that MRI can be safely performed at 3.0 T in patients with an LAA occluder device in place [43]. In contrast to CT MRI does not require radiation or iodinated contrast agents. However, MRI has important limitations which include: the spatial resolution is lower compared to CT and TEE and patients who are not able to perform adequate breath holds or those who do not have MRI-compatible pacemakers or defibrillators cannot be properly scanned.

3.3 Intraprocedural Imaging

2D and 3D TEE are the most important imaging modalities used to support angiography during a LAA closure procedure. TEE is used to guide TSP, to verify wire, catheter and sheath positions in the LA and the LAA, to aid in the placement and the delivery of the selected device, to confirm correct device position and absence of relevant peri-device leakages and to monitor for complications [44].

Although multiplanar 2D TEE is most commonly used for intraprocedural guidance, intracardiac echocardiography (ICE) has also been suggested as a feasible alternative to TEE [45–47] for guiding the LAA closure procedure, especially in patients who are not suitable for TEE imaging. This imaging modality has the advantage of avoiding general anesthesia or deep sedation because the ICE catheter is introduced via femoral vein access and placed either in the right atrium, the LA (requiring a double puncture in the interatrial septum), the coronary sinus or the main or left pulmonary artery. Limitations of ICE include the lack of multiplanar imaging with this modality and need for an interventionalist experienced with ICE in order to maneuver the catheter effectively. 3D capabilities are available but only with a very limited 3D volume size (22° × 90°) that does not allow for wide angle image acquisitions.

In addition to providing X-plane imaging, 3D TEE can provide views where guide catheters and LAA occlusion devices as well as the LAA and the interatrial septum can be observed in a single view and in relation to each other [48, 49]. Steering maneuvers and proper device alignment and deployment can be performed more easily by using 2D TEE and 3D TEE in combination.

Before the procedure starts, thrombi and pericardial effusion should again be excluded, the function of the MV and the patency of the LSPV should be evaluated and landing zone dimensions should be re-assessed and matched with angiographic measurements after acquisition in order to select an appropriate device size.

The procedural steps are similar for both device types.

3.3.1 Transseptal Puncture

As a coaxial entry into the LAA is preferred for optimal device positioning, the determination of the TSP site is of major importance (Fig. 3.12). As the course of the LAA is directed anteriorly and the ostium is either laterally or more anteriorly localized, the preferred puncture site is in the posterior region of the fossa ovalis. The superior-inferior position of the TSP is not as critical as the anterior-posterior, but a more inferior puncture site is generally preferable, especially when an Amulet device is chosen. The positioning of the transseptal needle starts usually by providing a long axis bi-caval view (~90–110°). In this view the retrieval of the sheath from the superior vena cava (SVC) downwards to the fossa is observed. Once the tip of the sheath reached the middle or the inferior part of the fossa (identified by a tent-like protrusion of the interatrial septum (IAS) with the tip of the “tent” pointing towards the LA), the anterior-posterior orientation needs to be verified in a short axis view (~45°). As shown in Fig. 3.12a, this imaging step is facilitated by using X-plane imaging which provides short axis and bi-caval (long axis) views simultaneously. Once a posterior and inferior position is adequately confirmed (lateral or

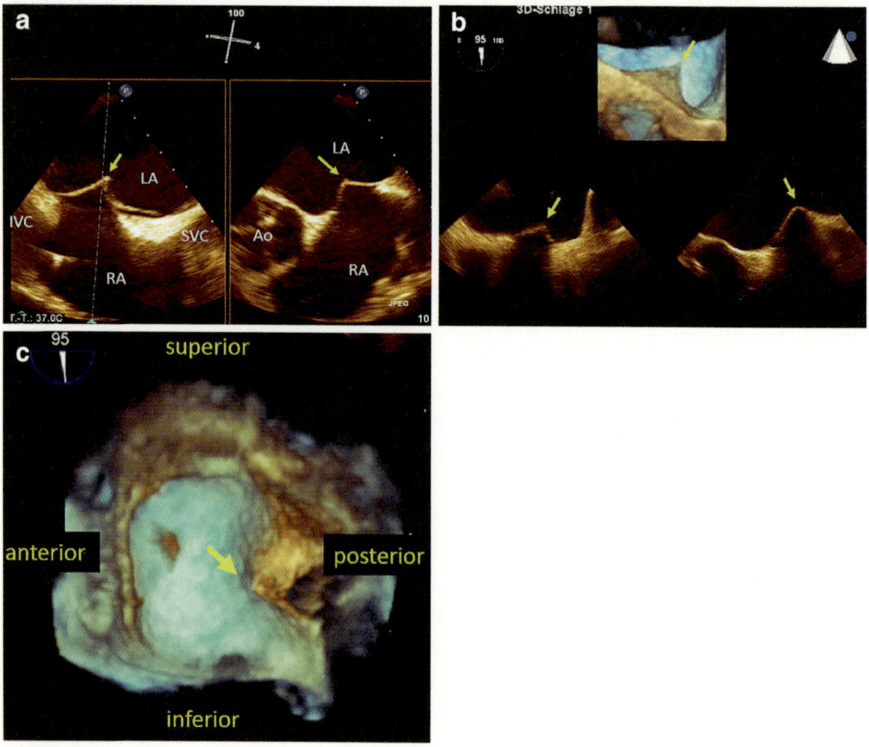

Fig. 3.12 **(a, b, c)** *Guidance of transseptal puncture*. (**a**) X-plane imaging facilitates the determination of the transseptal puncture site (marked with *yellow arrows*) by providing a bi-caval view (superior and inferior orientation; left image) and a short axis view (anterior-posterior orientation; right image) simultaneously. The "tenting" of the IAS should be clearly visible. In (**b**) the tenting of the IAS is seen in a lateral real-time 3D TEE view (*upper panel*) and in the corresponding bi-caval (*bottom left*) and short axis views (*bottom right*). In (**c**) a real-time 3D TEE enface view is used to confirm the transseptal puncture site in the posterior–inferior region of the fossa ovalis. The *yellow arrow head* marks the point of tenting by the transseptal needle just prior to puncture. LA = left atrium, RA = right atrium; IVC = inferior vena cava; SVC = superior vena cava; Ao = aorta; IAS = interatrial septum

enface 3D TEE views from the LA side can also be helpful in determining the preferred TSP site; Fig. 3.12b, c) the IAS can be punctured safely under continuous TEE control. A very mobile or stiff interatrial septum can cause difficulties, which may be addressed by crossing the interatrial septum with:

- the stiff end of a coronary wire,
- the needle stylet,
- diathermy,
- or radiofrequency puncture needles.

3.3.2 *Positioning of the Delivery Sheath and Device Deployment*

Once the septum is crossed a wire is positioned in the LSPV as seen in Fig. 3.13 and the delivery sheath is introduced into the LA. The crossing of the septum with the delivery sheath should be carefully monitored by TEE and fluoroscopy to ensure a smooth passage through the septum and proper orientation of the sheath. The sheath is then placed in the LSPV. This step is best imaged in short axis views in which the

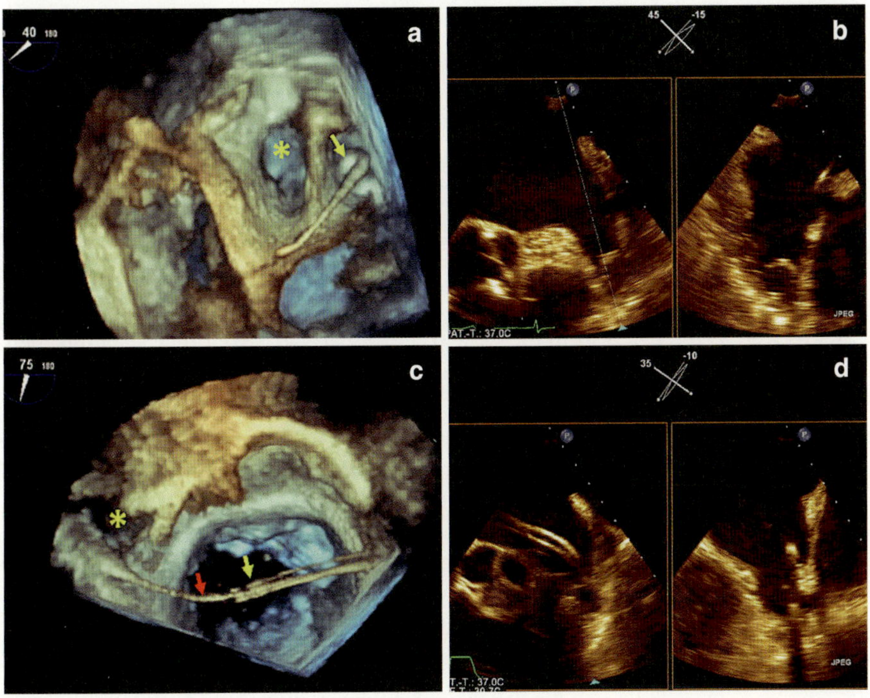

Fig. 3.13 (**a–d**) *Procedural steps*. In (**a**) the confirmation of the wire position in the left superior pulmonary vein (LSPV) (*yellow arrow*) is shown in an enface 3D TEE view. The left atrial appendage (LAA) is marked with a *yellow asterisk*. In (**b**) the correct position of the pigtail catheter (*yellow arrows*) is confirmed in a X-plane view. (**c**) illustrates the coaxial introduction of the delivery sheath (*yellow arrow*) over the pigtail catheter (*red arrow*) into the LAA (*yellow asterisk*) in a 3D enface view and in (**d**) the positioning of the sheath within the LAA is observed again in a X-plane view. (**e**) On the left side the position of the lobe of an Amulet device can be seen in a 3D TEE enface view. The stepwise development of the disc is then illustrated in the next images until the disc is fully deployed (*right*). In (**f**) a gentle, continuous tug test is shown to confirm the stability of the device. It is important, that the distal lobe remains in the same position. In (**g**) the appearance of a flattend "roman helmet" of the lobe after positioning can be appreciated (*yellow dotted line*) best in a fluoroscopic image

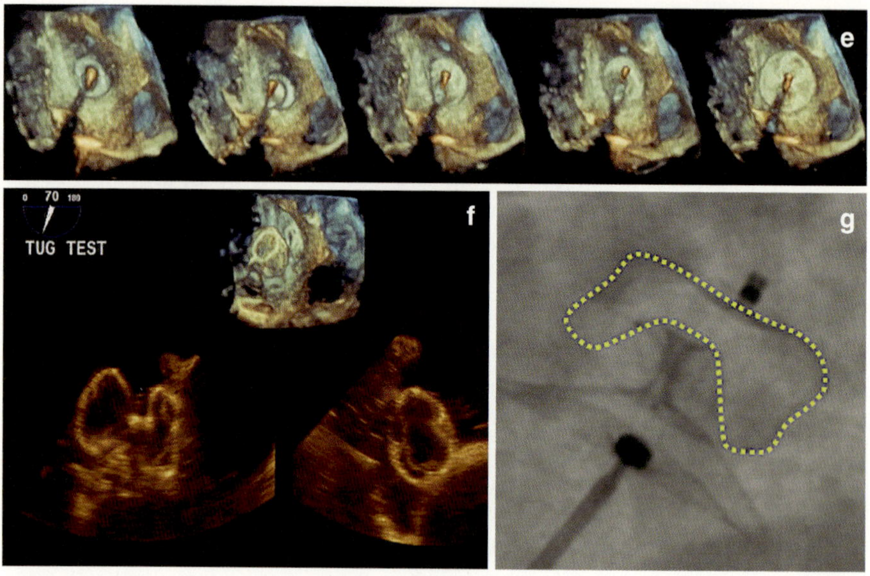

Fig. 3.13 (continued)

LAA as well as the LSPV is in the view (typically at ~45°–70°). The sheath is then retrieved over the Coumadin ridge and directed towards the LAA orifice.

For the introduction of the delivery system into the LAA X-plane imaging (simultaneous short axis view at ~ 45° and long axis view at ~135°) is helpful to confirm coaxial sheath alignment. The delivery sheath is usually introduced into the LAA over a soft, protective pigtail catheter (Fig. 3.13) (experienced operators may do this maneuver without the protection given by a pigtail catheter when an Amulet device is used provided that the TEE imaging quality offers appropriate guidance and it is not necessary to enter the LAA very deeply).

When a Watchman device is used the depth of the delivery sheath within the LAA cavity is determined by the selected device size and the anatomical features that define the landing zone. Markers on the delivery sheath are visible on TEE when the sheath is coaxially aligned. These markers are also visible on fluoroscopy and allow for an anatomical correlation of both imaging modalities. As the introduction of the Watchman device into the delivery sheath may straighten the sheath thus affecting the distal sheath position in the LAA this step must be carefully monitored, preferably again in simultaneous 45° and 135° X-plane views. After re-confirmation of the correct positioning of the sheath, the pigtail catheter is removed and the device is deployed.

When an Amulet device is used the tip of the delivery sheath is positioned approximately 10–15 mm beyond the level of the LCx in the LAA cavity in accordance with the pre-defined landing zone for the lobe of the device. The lobe is then entered, and if the position within the lobe is satisfactory, the disc is deployed as demonstrated in Fig. 3.13.

3.3.3 Assessment of the Final Result

Complete closure of the LAA without any interfering with or altering neighboring structures (namely the MV and the LSPV) is the principle purpose of the procedure and should be assessed immediately after device placement by the use of fluoroscopy (complete closure is confirmed by the administration of contrast agents) and 2D and 3D TEE. Color-flow Doppler with a low Nyquist limit (~30 cm/s) allows for the evaluation of low flow around the device and within the LAA cavity (as the Watchman device functions as a filter, visible flow on the LAA side of the device and within the LAA cavity is a normal finding after implantation as long as a relevant peri-device leak can be excluded. The exclusion of the LAA from the systemic circulation will be completed, when the device is endothelialized (Fig. 3.14)). For peri-device flow with higher velocity jets a Nyquist limit around 50 cm/s may be adequate. A residual leak with a jet size ≤5 mm seems acceptable, as this criterion was associated with non-inferiority in the device group compared to warfarin therapy in the PROTECT- AF-trial [50]. Damage or distortion of the MV or the LSPV is best imaged by using an enface 3D view.

A correct device position is of major importance. In case the device is positioned too deep into the cavity of the LAA, more proximally located lobes may stay uncovered. On the other hand, when a device is positioned too proximal it may not be adequately compressed and therefore unstable with an increased risk of device migration or embolization.

Therefore, specific device release criteria for each of the devices should be assessed carefully as they minimize the risk of complications. Generally, the final assessment should be made again in 0°, 45°, 90° and 135° imaging planes.

When a Watchman device is implanted, the release criteria can be summarized with the acronym "**PASS**" which is standing for:

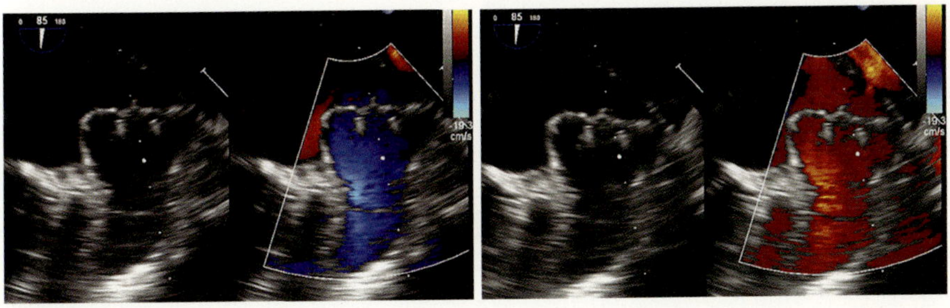

Fig. 3.14 *Assessment of peri- device leakage after implantation of a Watchman occluder.* A low pulse repetition frequency (19 cm/s) is used to assess for peri- device flow. No leak next to the device can be seen, bút as the Watchman device functions like a filter, flow through the device can be observed in atrial diastole (*left*) and systole (*right*)

Position: the device should be positioned symmetrically in the center of the LAA slightly below the LAA ostium or at the ostial plane. The device should not protrude >4–7 mm beyond the LAA ostium depending on the device size as outlined in the manufacturer's instructions for use (the most critical region is the posterior part of the LAA ostium which has to be evaluated in the 135° view).

Anchoring: fixations hooks should be in contact with the LAA wall (Fig. 3.15). A tug test is often used to confirm stability of device placement (see text below).

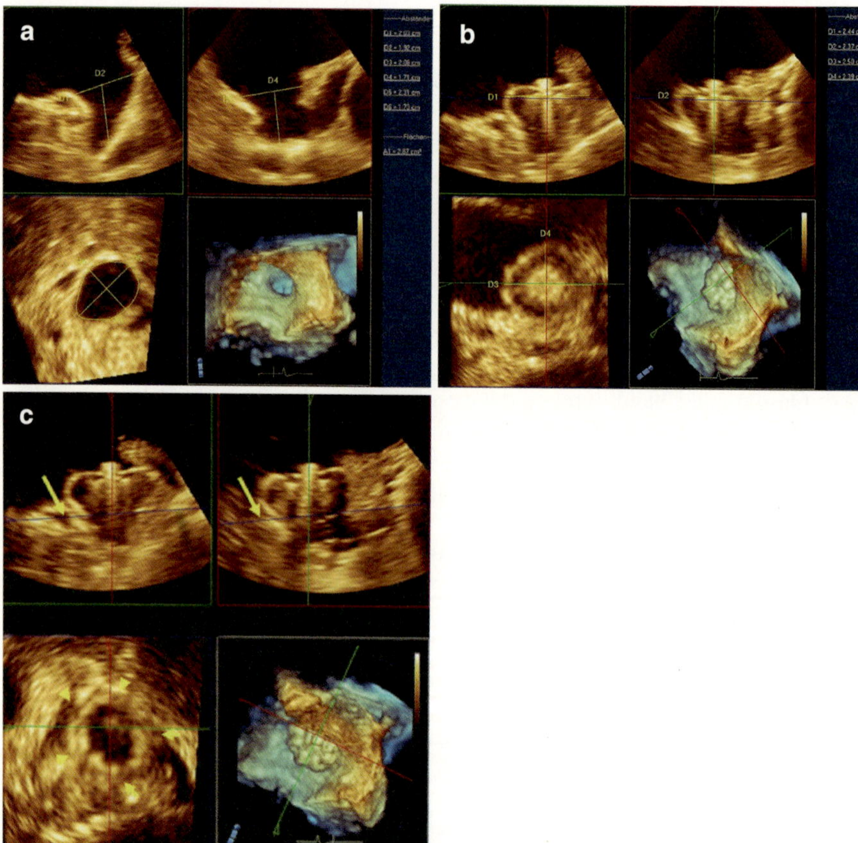

Fig. 3.15 (**a**, **b**, **c**) *Final device position and measurement of compression after implantation of a Watchman device*. (**a**) Measurement of the landing zone parameter by using 3D TEE cropping tools. The largest diameter is measured pre-procedurally in the Z-plane (23.1 mm; *red double arrow*; *bottom left*;). Accordingly, a 27 mm device was chosen. (**b**) After implantation the compression was measured in different planes (The screw should be visible in all images for this measurements- otherwise the device would be measured off-axis). Device measurements ranged between 23.7 and 25 mm. Compression therefore ranged from 8%–12%. The final position of the Watchman device can be assessed in b in a 45°, 135° (*upper left* and *upper right*) in a Z-plane (*bottom left*) and in a 3D enface view (*bottom right*). In (**c**) the *blue cropping line* (*yellow arrows*) is placed at the level of the hooks. In the corresponding Z-plane (*bottom left*) the entire circumference at this level can be judged and the contact to the LAA wall can be evaluated in detail. The *yellow arrow head* marks the point of measurement for device expansion

Sealing: a peri-device leak >5 mm must be excluded.

Size: a device compression of at least 8–20% of the original device size has to be confirmed. Some others recommend a higher compression of 15–30% (we are in agreement) (Fig. 3.15).

To fulfill the device release criteria for the Amulet device it is required that two-thirds of the lobe are positioned distal to the LCx. Some amount of compression should be visible on the lobe which usually has the appearance of a flat "roman helmet" (Fig. 3.13). The disc should cover and seal the LAA ostium with a concave shape and the waist in between the lobe and the disc should be clearly visible. The fixation anchors should be engaged to the LAA wall. In addition, after confirmation of the release criteria a gentle traction ("tugtest") that is applied to the device should demonstrate a stable device position. During this tugtest the device and the surrounding LAA tissue should move in unison and the position of the device should not change during this maneuver (Fig. 3.13).

In case of an unstable or suboptimal device position, the occluders can be retracted and re-deployed in most of the cases (complete retrieval into the sheath is not recommended for the Amulet device). After the final device assessment and before the TEE probe is removed, the patient should be re-assessed for any fluid in the pericardial space (a subcostal TTE view should be performed in addition in case there is any doubt) and the iatrogenic ASD after TSP should be evaluated and measured by 2D and 3D TEE imaging with and without color Doppler in order to provide a bench mark for further follow-up.

3.3.4 Monitoring of Complications

Complications may occur acutely at any time during a LAA closure procedure (Fig. 3.16) or delayed during patient follow-up (Fig. 3.17). In order to avoid or at least to minimize serious clinical consequences, complications have to be detected immediately after occurence by the use of echocardiography.

Pericardial effusion or tamponade may occur due to an incorrect TSP or due to a perforation of the LA or the LAA by wires, catheters or the device itself [50–53]. The interventionalist should be prepared to perform a pericardial drainage and in some cases surgery may be required.

Device embolization due to incorrect sizing or suboptimal device deployment occurs in 0–2.7% with different devices [50, 54–56]. Transcatheter removal e.g. by the use of snares/forceps may be attempted. If device retrieval is not successful, surgery will be necessary.

Thrombus formation on interventional instruments or on the device can occur acutely during the intervention or delayed (incidence generally around 5% [50, 54, 57]). The thrombus usually resolves with anticoagulation therapy.

Residual peri-device flow into the LAA is a very common finding but does not appear to be associated with an increased risk of stroke provided that the leak measures <5 mm in width [50]. The risk of relevant peri-device leaks may be minimized by careful sizing and an adequate morphological assessment before device implantation.

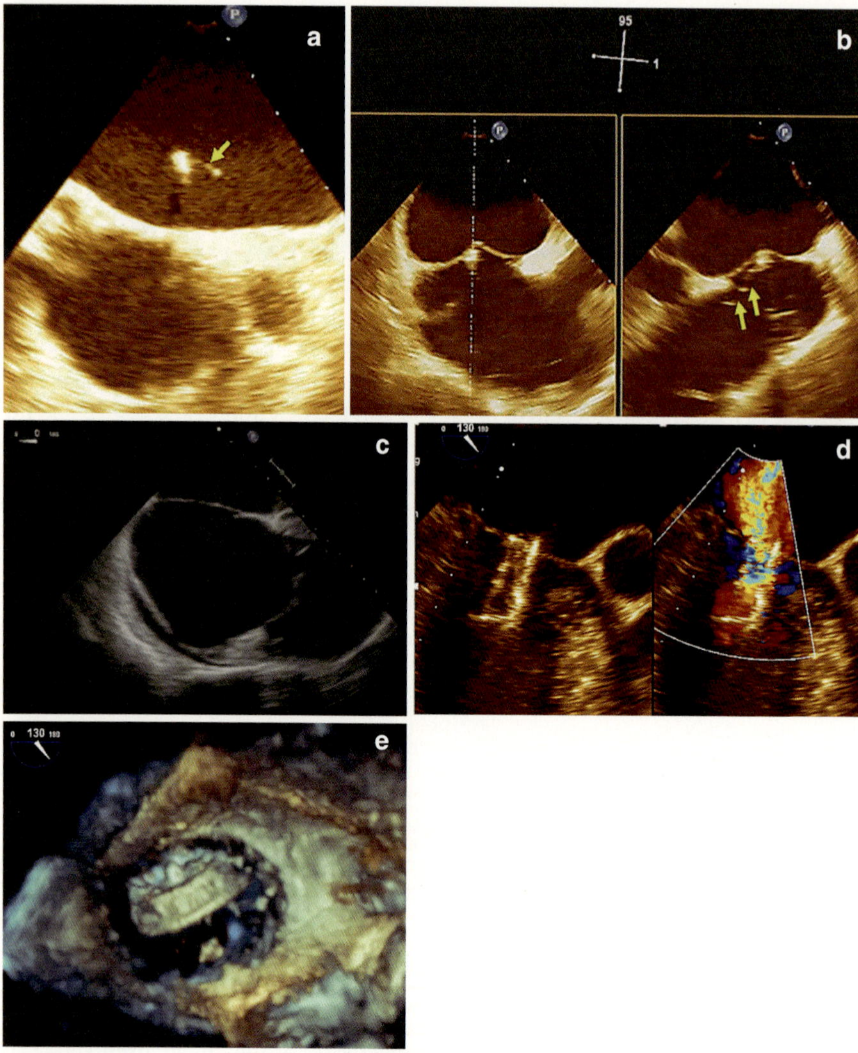

Fig. 3.16 (**a**–**e**) *Intraprocedural complications*: in (**a**) a thrombus can be observed that is attached to the sheath on the left atrial side (*yellow arrow*). In (**b**) a filiform thrombus that is attached to a SL1 needle can be seen (*yellow arrows*). (**c**) shows fluid in the pericardial space and in (**d**) a 2D TEE long axis view at 130° with and without color Doppler shows an embolized Amplatzer Cardiac Plug device that is caught in the mitral valve apparatus thus causing severe mitral regurgitation. In (**e**) the embolized device can be seen in a 3 D enface view in the LV from a left atrial aspect (mitral valve tissue cannot be seen due to the lowered gain)

Because of the close anatomical relationship a device placed in the LAA cavity can potentially cause left superior pulmonary vein obstruction or alter the MV apparatus or the LCx, but to our knowledge no cases describing one of these potential complications have been reported to date (June 2016).

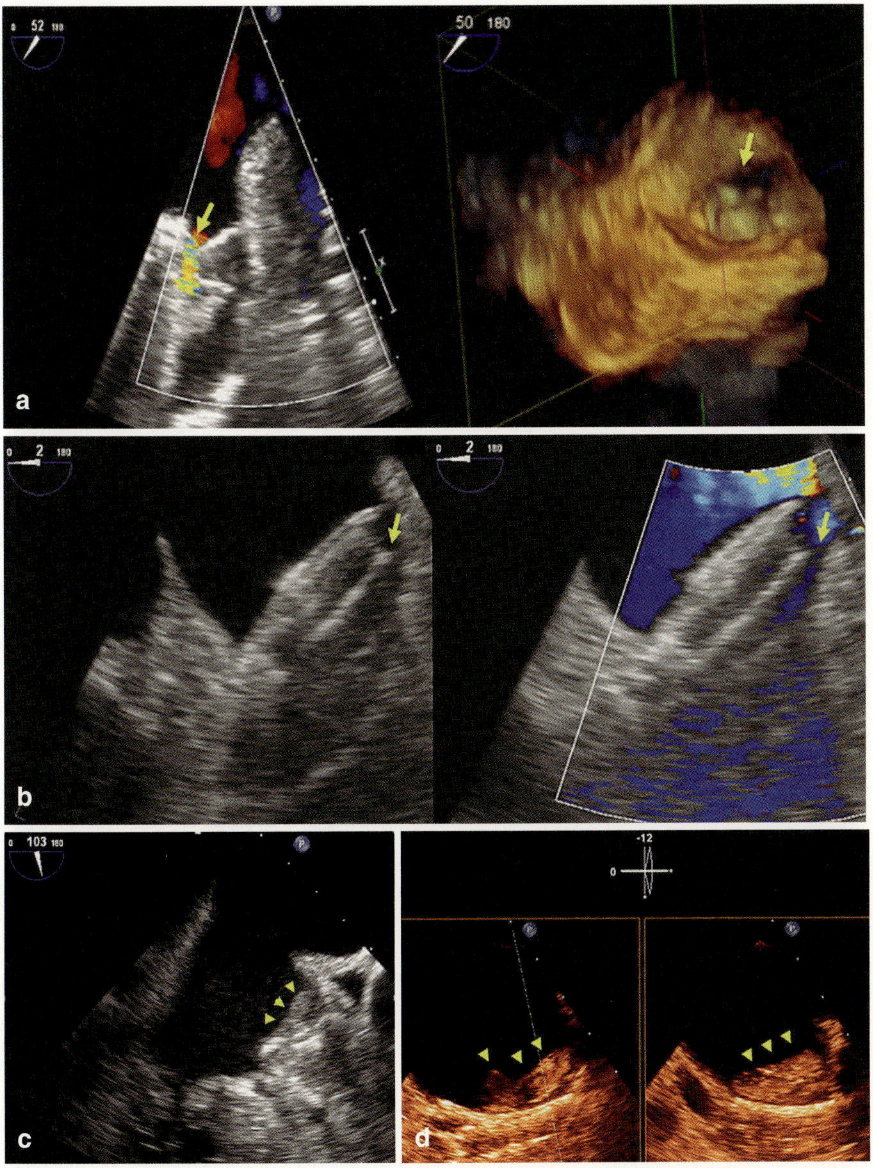

Fig. 3.17 (**a**–**d**) *Complications during follow-up*: in (**a**) peri-device leakage (*yellow arrows*) can be identified due to an uncovered lobe in medial location in a 52° 2D TEE view with color Doppler (*left*) and in a 3D TEE enface view (*right*). The device is undersized and the distal struts are caught in the main LAA lobe which is positioned laterally. (**b**) gives an example of a peri-device leakage in 2D TEE without (*left*) and with (*right*) color Doppler next to an Amplatzer Cardiac Plug. This device has no contact to the cranial LAA wall. No compression can be seen on the lobe and the disc shows a convex shape. In (**c**) a thrombus on the left atrial side of a Watchman device is shown and in (**d**) and a thrombus on the left atrial side of an Amplatzer Cardiac Plug device can be seen in a X-plane image (*yellow arrowheads*).

3.4 Post-Procedural Imaging

Before the patient is discharged from the hospital after a LAA closure procedure a TTE should be performed to confirm that there has been no relevant device migration, no new pericardial effusion has developed and there has been no increase in the size of a small pericardial effusion (if present earlier).

There is no consensus on when best to perform serial follow-up investigations, but TEE is often used initially between 45 days and 3–4 months post-procedure to exclude thrombus formation at the device and confirm sealing. Many centers continue with aspirin monotherapy or no therapy once complete closure and absence of thrombus formation has been confirmed. Further standard echocardiographic follow-up's may be performed at 6 and 12 months. In case no device migration or complications have occurred after one year following implantation, further surveillance is then performed annually by using TTE in most institutions. Abnormalities detected by TTE should be studied by an additional TEE for clarification.

During each follow-up visit the device is re-assessed for a stable and unchanged position, erosion, thrombus formation and peri- device leakages. Notably, it has been demonstrated that intra-procedural leaks can increase in size over time and persist over a year. New leaks may occur during follow-up due to remodeling processes [58]. In some patients with a relevant persistent leak due to an uncovered lobe, the implantation of a second device may be an option to complete LAA coverage [59–61].

References

1. Su P, McCarthy KP, Ho SY. Occluding the left atrial appendage: anatomical considerations. Heart. 2008;94:1166–70.
2. Sanchez-Quintana D, Cabrera JA, Climent V, Farre J, Weiglein A, Ho SY. How close are the phrenic nerves to cardiac structures? Implications for cardiac interventionalists. J Cardiovasc Electrophysiol. 2005;16:309–13.
3. Veinot JP, Harrity PJ, Gentile F, et al. Anatomy of the normal left atrial appendage: a quantitative study of age-related changes in 500 autopsy hearts: implications for echocardiographic examination. Circulation. 1997;96:3112–5.
4. Lopez-Minguez JR, Gonzalez-Fernandez R, Fernandez-Vegas C, et al. Anatomical classification of left atrial appendages in specimens applicable to CT imaging techniques for implantation of amplatzer cardiac plug. J Cardiovasc Electrophysiol. 2014;25:976–84.
5. Schwinger ME, Gindea AJ, Freedberg RS, Kronzon I. The anatomy of the interatrial septum: a transesophageal echocardiographic study. Am Heart J. 1990;119:1401–5.
6. Shirani J, Alaeddini J. Structural remodeling of the left atrial appendage in patients with chronic non-valvular atrial fibrillation: implications for thrombus formation, systemic embolism, and assessment by transesophageal echocardiography. Cardiovasc Pathol. 2000;9:95–101.
7. Gage BF, van Walraven C, Pearce L, et al. Selecting patients with atrial fibrillation for anticoagulation: stroke risk stratification in patients taking aspirin. Circulation. 2004;110:2287–92.

8. Agmon Y, Khandheria BK, Gentile F, Seward JB. Echocardiographic assessment of the left atrial appendage. J Am Coll Cardiol. 1999;34:1867–77.
9. Manning WJ, Weintraub RM, Waksmonski CA, et al. Accuracy of transesophageal echocardiography for identifying left atrial thrombi. A prospective, intraoperative study. Ann Intern Med. 1995;123:817–22.
10. Beigel R, Wunderlich NC, Ho SY, Arsanjani R, Siegel RJ. The left atrial appendage: anatomy, function, and noninvasive evaluation. JACC Cardiovasc Imaging. 2014;7:1251–65.
11. Marek D, Vindis D, Kocianova E. Real time 3-dimensional transesophageal echocardiography is more specific than 2-dimensional TEE in the assessment of left atrial appendage thrombosis. Biomed Pap Med Fac Univ Palacky Olomouc Czech Repub. 2013;157:22–6.
12. Maltagliati A, Pepi M, Tamborini G, et al. Usefulness of multiplane transesophageal echocardiography in the recognition of artifacts and normal anatomical variants that may mimic left atrial thrombi in patients with atrial fibrillation. Ital Heart J. 2003;4:797–802.
13. Anwar A, Nosir YM, Ajam A, Chamsi-Pasha H. Central role of real-time three-dimensional echocardiography in the assessment of intracardiac thrombi. Int J Cardiovasc Imaging. 2010;26:519–26.
14. Muller S, Feuchtner G, Bonatti J et al. Value of transesophageal 3D echocardiography as an adjunct to conventional 2D imaging in preoperative evaluation of cardiac masses. Echocardiography 2008;25:624–31.
15. Asch FM, Bieganski SP, Panza JA, Weissman NJ. Real-time 3-dimensional echocardiography evaluation of intracardiac masses. Echocardiography. 2006;23:218–24.
16. Ahmed S, Nanda NC, Miller AP, et al. Volume quantification of intracardiac mass lesions by transesophageal three-dimensional echocardiography. Ultrasound Med Biol. 2002;28:1389–93.
17. Habib G, Lancellotti P, Antunes MJ, et al. 2015 ESC Guidelines for the management of infective endocarditis: the task force for the management of infective endocarditis of the European Society of Cardiology (ESC) endorsed by: European Association for Cardio-Thoracic Surgery (EACTS), the European Association of Nuclear Medicine (EANM). Eur Heart J. 2015;36:3075–128.
18. Donal E, Yamada H, Leclercq C, Herpin D. The left atrial appendage, a small, blind-ended structure: a review of its echocardiographic evaluation and its clinical role. Chest. 2005;128:1853–62.
19. Chan SK, Kannam JP, Douglas PS, Manning WJ. Multiplane transesophageal echocardiographic assessment of left atrial appendage anatomy and function. Am J Cardiol. 1995;76:528–30.
20. Freixa X, Tzikas A, Basmadjian A, Garceau P, Ibrahim R. The chicken-wing morphology: an anatomical challenge for left atrial appendage occlusion. J Interv Cardiol. 2013;26:509–14.
21. Tzikas A, Gafoor S, Meerkin D, et al. Left atrial appendage occlusion with the AMPLATZER Amulet device: an expert consensus step-by-step approach. EuroIntervention. 2016;11:1512–21.
22. Onalan O, Crystal E. Left atrial appendage exclusion for stroke prevention in patients with nonrheumatic atrial fibrillation. Stroke. 2007;38:624–30.
23. Stollberger C, Schneider B, Finsterer J. Serious complications from dislocation of a Watchman left atrial appendage occluder. J Cardiovasc Electrophysiol. 2007;18:880–1.
24. Spencer RJ, DeJong P, Fahmy P, et al. Changes in left atrial appendage dimensions following volume loading during percutaneous left atrial appendage closure. J Am Coll Cardiol Intv. 2015;8:1935–41.
25. Shah SJ, Bardo DM, Sugeng L, et al. Real-time three-dimensional transesophageal echocardiography of the left atrial appendage: initial experience in the clinical setting. J Am Soc Echocardiogr. 2008;21:1362–8.
26. Nucifora G, Faletra FF, Regoli F, et al. Evaluation of the left atrial appendage with real-time 3-dimensional transesophageal echocardiography: implications for catheter-based left atrial appendage closure. Circ Cardiovasc Imaging. 2011;4:514–23.

27. Nakajima H, Seo Y, Ishizu T, et al. Analysis of the left atrial appendage by three-dimensional transesophageal echocardiography. Am J Cardiol. 2010;106:885–92.
28. Unsworth B, Sutaria N, Davies DW, Kanagaratnam P. Successful placement of left atrial appendage closure device is heavily dependent on 3-dimensional transesophageal imaging. J Am Coll Cardiol. 2011;58:1283.
29. Meier B, Blaauw Y, Khattab AA, et al. EHRA/EAPCI expert consensus statement on catheter-based left atrial appendage occlusion. Europace. 2014;16(10):1397–416.
30. Ismail TF, Panikker S, Markides V, et al. CT imaging for left atrial appendage closure: a review and pictorial essay. J Cardiovasc Comput Tomogr. 2015;9:89–102.
31. Martinez MW, Kirsch J, Williamson EE, et al. Utility of nongated multidetector computed tomography for detection of left atrial thrombus in patients undergoing catheter ablation of atrial fibrillation. JACC Cardiovasc Imaging. 2009;2:69–76.
32. Gottlieb I, Pinheiro A, Brinker JA, et al. Diagnostic accuracy of arterial phase 64-slice multi-detector CT angiography for left atrial appendage thrombus in patients undergoing atrial fibrillation ablation. J Cardiovasc Electrophysiol. 2008;19:247–51.
33. van Rosendael PJ, Katsanos S, van den Brink OW, et al. Geometry of left atrial appendage assessed with multidetector-row computed tomography: implications for transcatheter closure devices. EuroIntervention. 2014;10:364–71.
34. Wang Y, Di Biase L, Horton RP, Nguyen T, Morhanty P, Natale A. Left atrial appendage studied by computed tomography to help planning for appendage closure device placement. J Cardiovasc Electrophysiol. 2010;21:973–82.
35. Di Biase L, Santangeli P, Anselmino M, et al. Does the left atrial appendage morphology correlate with the risk of stroke in patients with atrial fibrillation? Results from a multicenter study. J Am Coll Cardiol. 2012;60:531–8.
36. Khurram IM, Dewire J, Mager M, et al. Relationship between left atrial appendage morphology and stroke in patients with atrial fibrillation. Heart Rhythm. 2013;10:1843–9.
37. Jaguszewski M, Manes C, Puippe G, et al. Cardiac CT and echocardiographic evaluation of peri-device flow after percutaneous left atrial appendage closure using the AMPLATZER cardiac plug device. Catheter Cardiovasc Interv. 2015;85:306–12.
38. Ohyama H, Hosomi N, Takahashi T, et al. Comparison of magnetic resonance imaging and transesophageal echocardiography in detection of thrombus in the left atrial appendage. Stroke; a journal of cerebral circulation. 2003;34:2436–9.
39. Rathi VK, Reddy ST, Anreddy S, et al. Contrast-enhanced CMR is equally effective as TEE in the evaluation of left atrial appendage thrombus in patients with atrial fibrillation undergoing pulmonary vein isolation procedure. Heart Rhythm. 2013;10:1021–7.
40. Akoum N, Fernandez G, Wilson B, McGann C, Kholmovski E, Marrouche N. Association of atrial fibrosis quantified using LGE-MRI with atrial appendage thrombus and spontaneous contrast on transesophageal echocardiography in patients with atrial fibrillation. J Cardiovasc Electrophysiol. 2013;24:1104–9.
41. Muellerleile K, Sultan A, Groth M, et al. Velocity encoded cardiovascular magnetic resonance to assess left atrial appendage emptying. J Cardiovasc Magn Reson. 2012;14:39.
42. Mohrs OK, Wunderlich N, Petersen SE, Pottmeyer A, Kauczor HU. Contrast-enhanced CMR in patients after percutaneous closure of the left atrial appendage: a pilot study. J Cardiovasc Magn Reson. 2011;13:33.
43. Levine GN, Gomes AS, Arai AE, et al. Safety of magnetic resonance imaging in patients with cardiovascular devices: an American Heart Association scientific statement from the Committee on Diagnostic and Interventional Cardiac Catheterization, Council on Clinical Cardiology, and the Council on Cardiovascular Radiology and Intervention: endorsed by the American College of Cardiology Foundation, the North American Society for Cardiac Imaging, and the Society for Cardiovascular Magnetic Resonance. Circulation. 2007;116:2878–91.
44. Wunderlich NC, Beigel R, Swaans MJ, Ho SY, Siegel RJ. Percutaneous interventions for left atrial appendage exclusion: options, assessment, and imaging using 2D and 3D echocardiography. JACC Cardiovasc Imaging. 2015;8:472–88.

45. MacDonald ST, Newton JD, Ormerod OJ. Intracardiac echocardiography off piste? Closure of the left atrial appendage using ICE and local anesthesia. Catheter Cardiovasc Interv. 2011;77:124–7.
46. Berti S, Paradossi U, Meucci F, et al. Periprocedural intracardiac echocardiography for left atrial appendage closure: a dual-center experience. JACC Cardiovasc Interv. 2014;7:1036–44.
47. Fassini G, Dello Russo A, Conti S, Tondo C. An alternative transseptal intracardiac echocardiography strategy to guide left atrial appendage closure: the first described case. J Cardiovasc Electrophysiol. 2014;25:1269–71.
48. Perk G, Lang RM, Garcia-Fernandez MA, et al. Use of real time three-dimensional transesophageal echocardiography in intracardiac catheter based interventions. J Am Soc Echocardiogr. 2009;22:865–82.
49. Lang RM, Badano LP, Tsang W, et al. EAE/ASE recommendations for image acquisition and display using three-dimensional echocardiography. J Am Soc Echocardiogr. 2012;25:3–46.
50. Holmes DR, Reddy VY, Turi ZG, et al. Percutaneous closure of the left atrial appendage versus warfarin therapy for prevention of stroke in patients with atrial fibrillation: a randomised non-inferiority trial. Lancet. 2009;374:534–42.
51. Price MJ, Gibson DN, Yakubov SJ, et al. Early safety and efficacy of percutaneous left atrial appendage suture ligation: results from the U.S. transcatheter LAA ligation consortium. J Am Coll Cardiol. 2014;64:565–72.
52. Reddy VY, Doshi SK, Sievert H, et al. Percutaneous left atrial appendage closure for stroke prophylaxis in patients with atrial fibrillation: 2.3-year follow-up of the PROTECT AF (Watchman left atrial appendage system for embolic protection in patients with atrial fibrillation) trial. Circulation. 2013;127:720–9.
53. Park JW, Bethencourt A, Sievert H, et al. Left atrial appendage closure with Amplatzer cardiac plug in atrial fibrillation: initial European experience. Catheter Cardiovasc Interv. 2011;77:700–6.
54. Reddy VY, Holmes D, Doshi SK, Neuzil P, Kar S. Safety of percutaneous left atrial appendage closure: results from the Watchman left atrial appendage system for embolic protection in patients with AF (PROTECT AF) clinical trial and the continued access registry. Circulation. 2011;123:417–24.
55. Lam YY, Yip GW, Yu CM, et al. Left atrial appendage closure with AMPLATZER cardiac plug for stroke prevention in atrial fibrillation: initial Asia-Pacific experience. Catheter Cardiovasc Interv. 2012;79:794–800.
56. Tzikas A, Shakir S, Gafoor S, et al. Left atrial appendage occlusion for stroke prevention in atrial fibrillation: multicentre experience with the AMPLATZER Cardiac Plug. EuroIntervention. 2015;10
57. Main ML, Fan D, Reddy VY, et al. Assessment of device-related thrombus and associated clinical outcomes with the WATCHMAN left atrial appendage closure device for embolic protection in patients with atrial fibrillation (from the PROTECT-AF Trial). Am J Cardiol. 2016;117:1127–34.
58. Freixa X, Tzikas A, Sobrino A, Chan J, Basmadjian AJ, Ibrahim R. Left atrial appendage closure with the Amplatzer Cardiac Plug: impact of shape and device sizing on follow-up leaks. Int J Cardiol. 2013;168:1023–7.
59. Wunderlich N, Wilson N, Sievert H. A novel approach to treat residual peridevice leakage after left-atrial appendage closure. Catheter Cardiovasc Interv. 2013;82:313–9.
60. Guerios EE, Gloekler S, Schmid M, Khattab A, Nietlispach F, Meier B. Double device left atrial appendage closure. EuroIntervention. 2015;11:470–6.
61. Hornung M, Gafoor S, Id D, et al. Catheter-based closure of residual leaks after percutaneous occlusion of the left atrial appendage. Catheter Cardiovasc Interv. 2016;87:1324–30.

Chapter 4
Access to the Left Atrium

4.1 Preparation of Transseptal Puncture

The technique of transseptal puncture is standardized and similar to the initial steps of pulmonary vein isolation as an antiarrhythmic therapy in atrial fibrillation or the preparation for a MitraClip procedure for mitral regurgitation. The right femoral vein is punctured ideally in a shallow angle following incision of the skin to allow the larger sheath needed for the device later on to pass skin and surrounding tissue easily. Many operators favor a SL1 sheath, where the Brockenbrough needle can be passed through the dilator. This allows to negotiate the fossa ovalis in a very controlled fashion (Fig. 5.3). In case of very dilated right atria as observed in heart failure patients additional pre-shaping of the Brockenbrough needle may be required. One has to notice that the SL1 wire 0.028 in. cannot be exchanged for the standard 0.034 in. J-wire. If the system doesn't allow for free rotation in the pelvic area because of a restrictive retroperitoneal space early decision for additional measures is recommended since even after transseptal puncture the device sheath (i.e. Watchman delivery sheath) must be rotated – this sheath is very soft; any resistance in the pelvic area will lead the sheath to torque and prevent any progress regarding the procedure. A 14F inner diameter TAVI sheath like i.e. the SJM sheath will allow to negotiate this problem. The SL1 sheath as well as the device sheath (Watchman or Amplatzer delivery sheath) can be easily introduced through this system (Fig. 4.1).

4.2 Puncture of the Fossa Ovalis

Advancing the SL1 sheath without a wire in place might be traumatic as the dilator plus needle might easily cross the fragile venous system. Once the SL1 sheath is placed into the superior vena cava and the wire is exchanged for the Brockenbrough needle, a pullback is performed until the systems falls into the fossa ovalis. A mid/posterior and inferior location for transseptal puncture is recommended to facilitate an

M.W. Bergmann et al., *Clinical Cases in LAA Occlusion*,
DOI 10.1007/978-3-319-51431-4_4

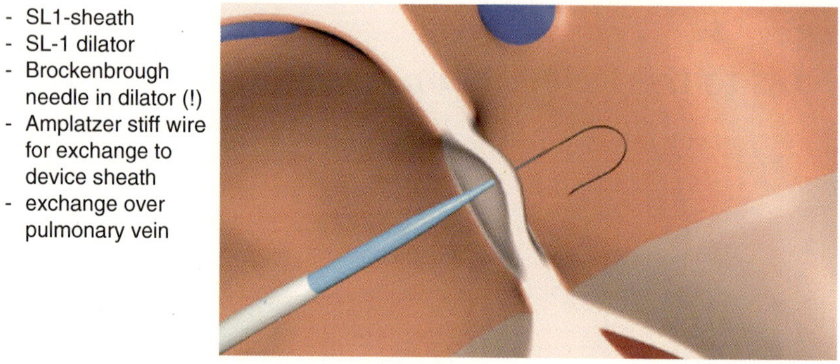

Fig. 4.1 Material for transseptal puncture: an SL1 sheath and its dilator equipped with a Brockenbrough needle allows to cross the Fossa ovalis. Shaping of the Brockenbrough needle does allow to negotiate also large atria where there is a difficulty to get close to the septum. For crossing the septum, the Brockenbrough needle is advanced slightly ("puncture") after tenting of the septum at the correct position with the dilator

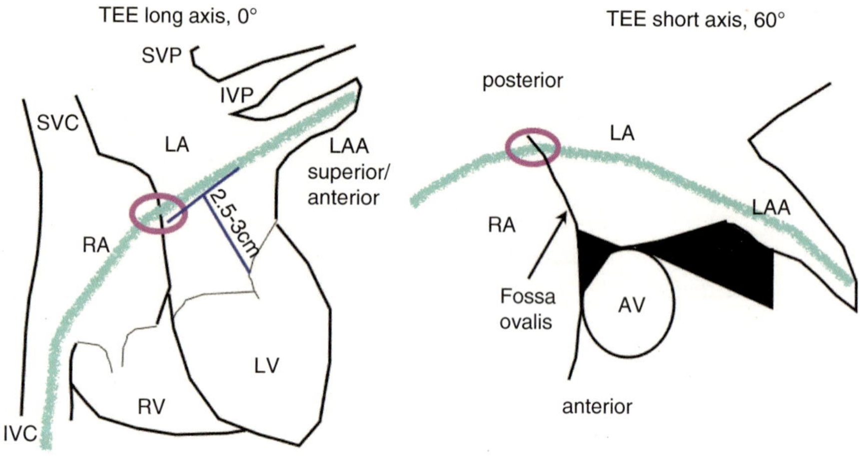

Fig. 4.2 Schematic view regarding the location of transseptal puncture inferior & posterior for easy, untorqued access to LAA

easy and straight access to the LAA (Fig. 5.4). The system should be pulled back with the needle in a 5 o'clock (to achieve a more posterior location: 7 o'clock) position (Figs. 5.5 and 5.6). Some operators position a pigtail catheter at the aortic valve in the noncoronary cusp – this serves as anatomic landmark where the needle should point to in both a RAO 30° and LAO 40° angiographic view (Fig. 5.7). Echocardiographic control of the location of septal tenting is recommended to verify an optimal position. Next the Brockenbrough needle is advance with a quick "puncture" movement. The sheath/dilator assembly follows; it is important to ensure that the sheath has crossed the interatrial septum prior to pull back the dilator and the needle. Echocardiographic monitoring of this step is highly recommended (Fig. 4.2).

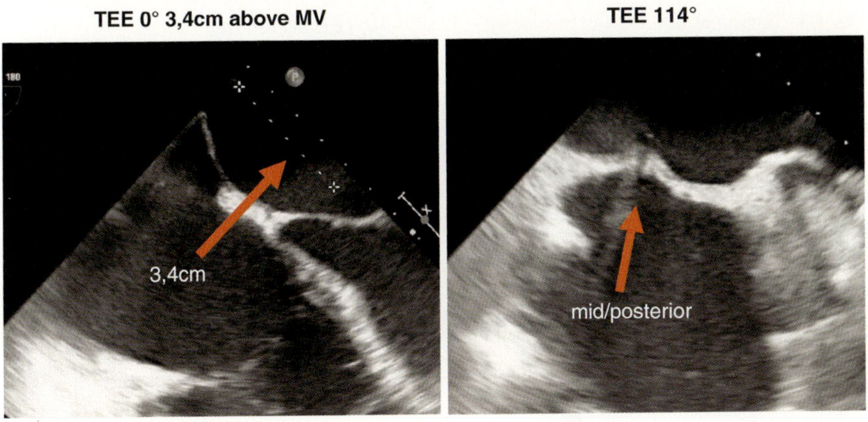

Fig. 4.3 Case 1: Tenting of the interatrial septum in two views prior to crossing the interatrial septum

4.3 Handling of Complications

Even if an appropriate tenting was seen prior to the "puncture" a dislocation of the transseptal needle due to a floppy septum or unexpected resistance may occur. Pressure monitoring following transseptal puncture allows to immediately recognize whether the sheath is positioned in the LA or has accidentally moved into the aorta or the epicardial space. In case of an accidental puncturing of the aorta (too anterior position) the needle can be retracted without complications in most cases as long as no larger sheath is introduced. In case of an epicardial location, the sheath should be left in space and a second SL1 system should be employed to finish the procedure. At the end of the procedure, pericardiac effusion has to be assessed to decide if a pigtail should be placed in the epicardial space before the dislocated sheath is pulled back (Fig. 4.3).

4.4 Technical Modifications of Left Atrium Access

With growing experience some operators use different approaches; although regarded as a compromise regarding sheath movement and access using a Persistent Foramen ovale for access has been done regularly by some centers and also lead to successful LAA closure. Sheath different to the standard SL1 are used by some operators. Dedicated devices including electropuncture are available to facilitate transseptal puncture in case of a very restrictive and thick septum (Figs. 4.4, 4.5 and 4.6).

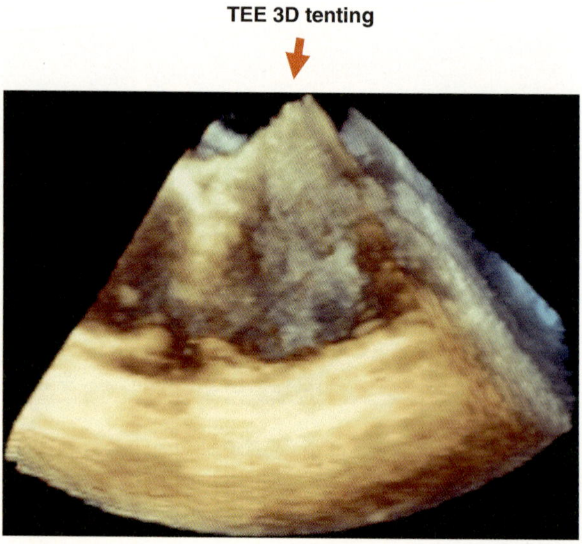

Fig. 4.4 Tenting of the interatrial septum at the fossa ovalis posterior/inferior just prior to puncture of the septum

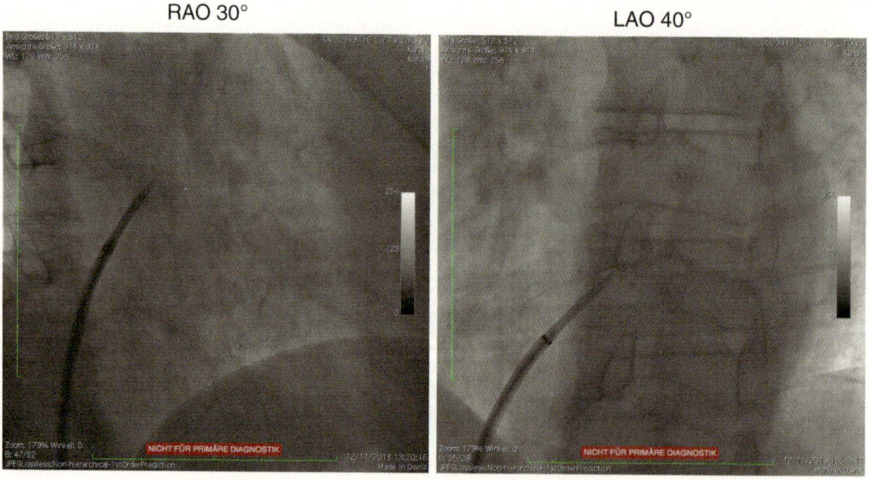

Fig. 4.5 Angiographic orientation of the SL1 sheath just prior to transseptal puncture. The Brockenbrough needle is orientated from 5 o'clock (normal heart) to 8 o'clock (dilated ventricle) in order to achieve a posterior puncture site

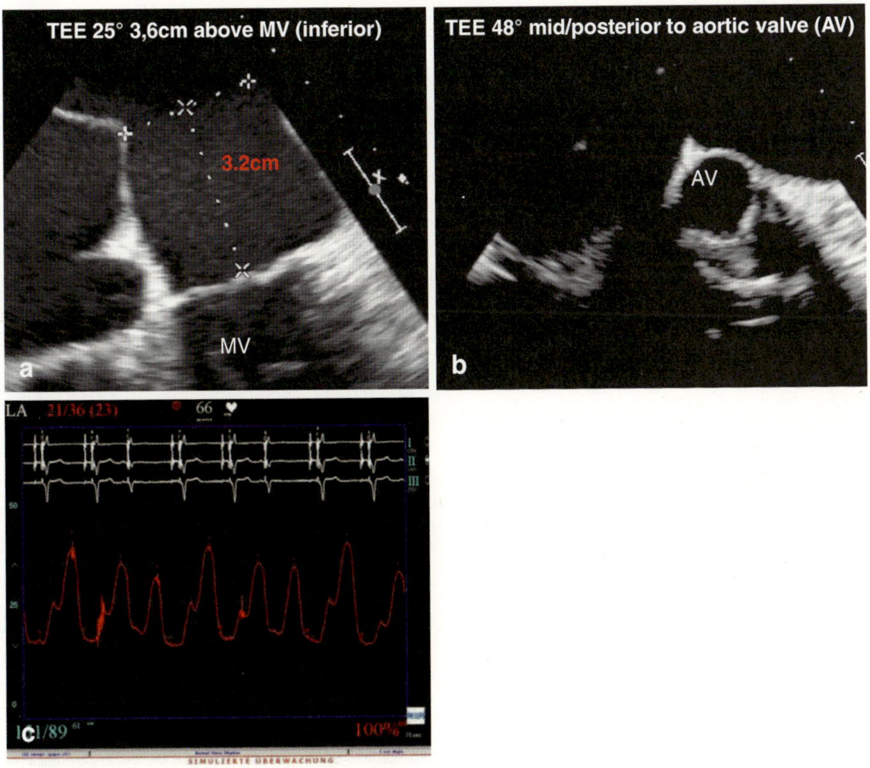

Fig. 4.6 Case 2: Location of transeptal puncture for LAA occlusion; visualization of tenting in long (**a**) and short (**b**) axis in TEE. Following transseptal puncture, left atrial pressure is monitored and documented (**c**)

Chapter 5
Practical Watchman Implantation

5.1 Device Features

The Watchman device consists of a nitinol frame with low radial force. It is available in five sizes (Fig. 5.1), which allow the occlusion of LAAs ranging from 16 mm to 30 mm as the largest diameter measured at the Watchman landing zone. In experienced hands, LAAs as small as 14 mm have been occluded without difficulties. LAA larger than 30 mm have been occluded employing the "kissing Watchman" technique. The following device characteristics are essential for successful closure:

- device anchoring is achieved by 10 flexible fixation barbs located at half the depth of the device just distal to the PET fabric
- PET covers the proximal 50% of device depth.
- PET fabric prevents thrombi from leaving the LAA immediately after release.
- PET fabric allows contrast to pass
- sheath is available in two shapes, "double curve" variant is the standard (Fig. 5.2)
- The Watchman sheath allows to measure depth by the radiopaque proximal rings (Fig. 5.2)
- Watchman landing zone is measured according to standardized anatomical landmarks. Compression of 20% has proven to be optimal for sealing and successful closure (Figs. 5.3, 5.4, 5.5 and 5.6)

Successful LAA closure is achieved with a step-by-step approach (Fig. 5.7). The device endothelializes over time until final coverage is achieved after around 3–6 months (Fig. 5.8). Antithrombotic treatment is recommend during this time with dual antiplatelet therapy (DAPT) being the most common choice in Europe whereas the PROTECT-AF Scheme (45 days of warfarin followed by DAPT until 6 months then aspirin alone) is the standard in the US. New data from the EWOLUTION registry point to the possibility of using NOAC during the first three months prior to switching to aspirin (Fig. 5.9).

M.W. Bergmann et al., *Clinical Cases in LAA Occlusion*,
DOI 10.1007/978-3-319-51431-4_5

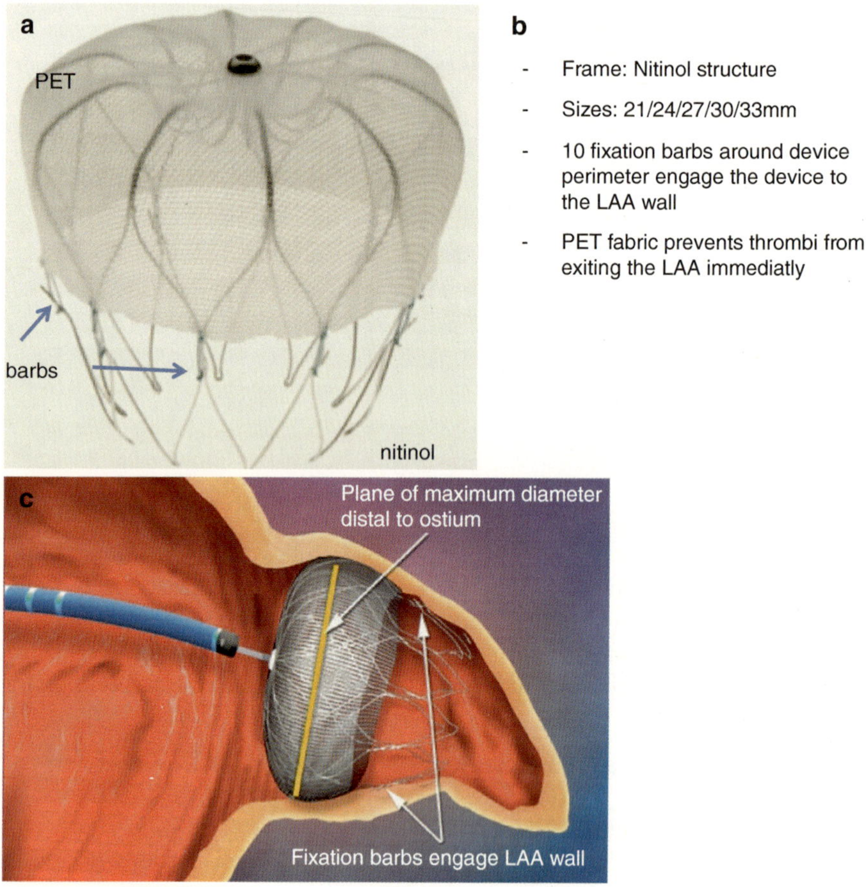

Fig. 5.1 The Watchman device consists of a nitinol structure covered with a PET (polyethyl terephthalate) cap of 160 micron filter (Fig. 5.1a). Ten fixation barbs around the middle part of the device perimeter engage the device to the LAA wall for anchoring. Available sizes are: 21, 24, 27, 30 and 33 mm (Fig. 5.1b, c)

5.2 Sheath Exchange

The access sheath and dilator are used to gain access to the LAA following a transseptal puncture. The Watchman sheath is available in two variations, the double curve (standard) and the single curve meant to have an easier access to a windsock type LAA (Fig. 5.2). In the early days of LAA occlusion, pericardial effusion both early and delayed was a quite common event that limited the benefit of this prophylactic intervention. It became clear that wire navigation of the fragile LAA and excessive device manipulation prior to device release is often responsible for this life threatening event to occur. Therefore exchange to the Watchman sheath over a stiff wire (Supracore 260 cm or Amplatzer stiff or super stiff 260 cm) located in the left superior pulmonary vein (LSPV) has been adopted as the default strategy as it

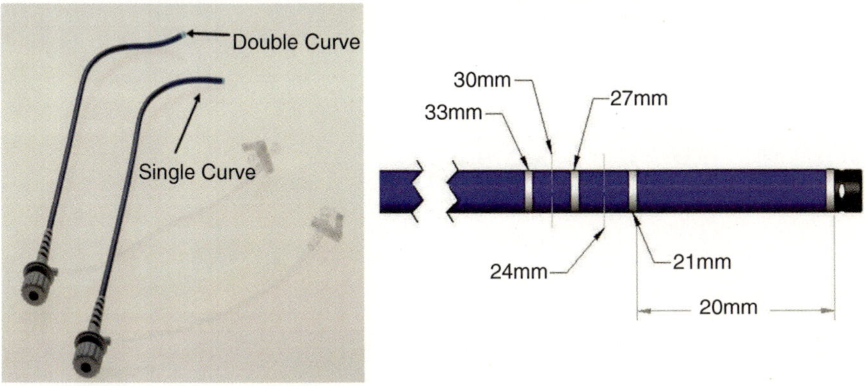

Fig. 5.2 Delivery sheaths for Watchman device implantation. Preformed curve shapes guide position into the LAA—most operators use the double curve sheath only. This sheath has an outer diameter of 14F (4.7 mm) and an inner diameter of 12F. The sheath has a working length of 75 cm allowing to use a standard pigtail catheter to negotiate the LAA. The distal markers allow to probe the depth of the LAA and are also useful for normalization of the angiographic measurements. The more proximal markers indicate the landing zone of the different device sizes: from distal to proximal the rings locate at appropriately the landing zone of the 21, 27 and 33 mm device. 24 and 30 are in between

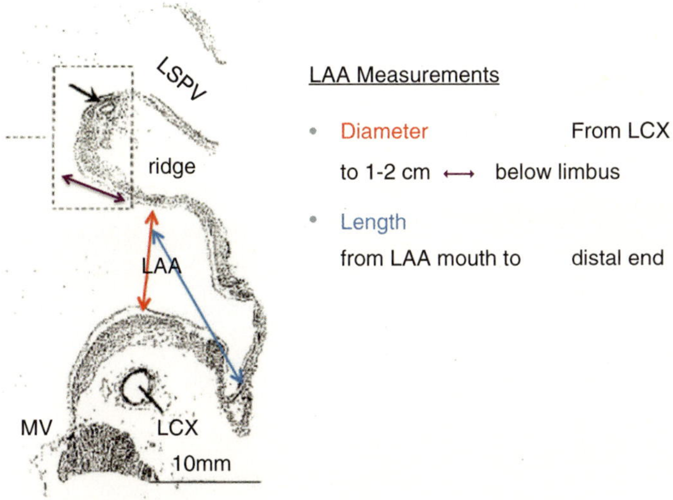

Fig. 5.3 Measurement of the Watchman landing zone diameter and the LAA depth. The proximal part of the ridge to the left superior pulmonary vein (LSPV) is considered to be part of the free left atrium (no trabecularization). The landing zone of the LAA for Watchman sizing is measured between the inferior tissue border close to the coronary circumflex artery visible in TEE. The superior part is located approximately 1–2 cm distal to the LSPV ridge orthogonal from the Cx tissue edge. Depth maybe measured along the visible axis, yet this is often not possible due to a 3D rotation of the LAA. Probing the depth with the Watchman sheath on the pigtail is recommended

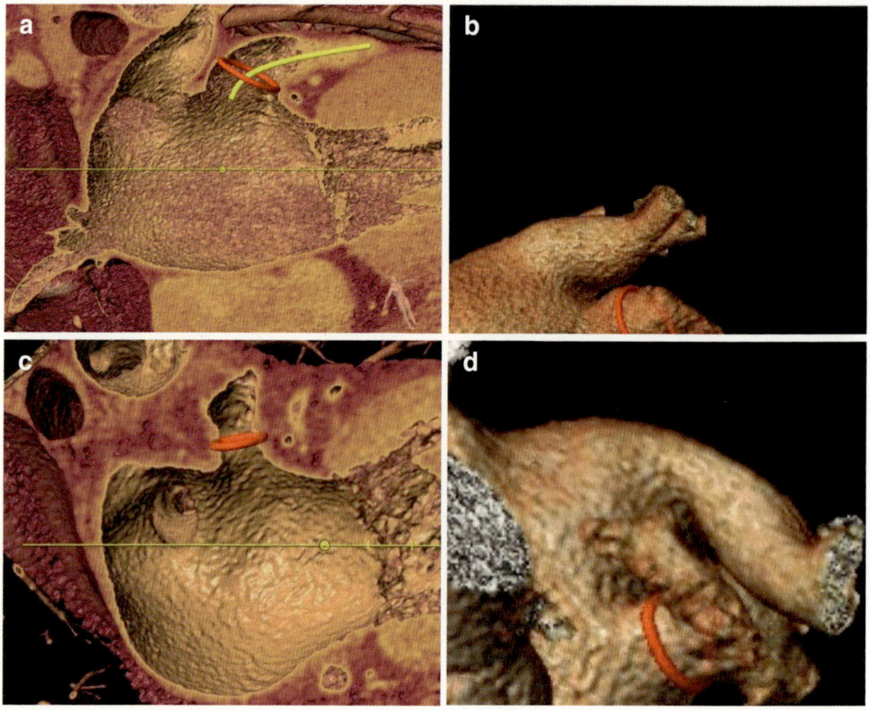

Fig. 5.4 Exemplary CT images of two patients illustrating the anatomic location of Watchman landing zone employed for correct sizing. (**a**, **b**) Internal and external imaging of a windsock LAA. Watchman landing zone diameters are measure from the Cx ridge to a point approx. 1–2 cm distal to the coumadin ridge. (**c**, **d**) Internal and external imaging of a classic chicken wing anatomy

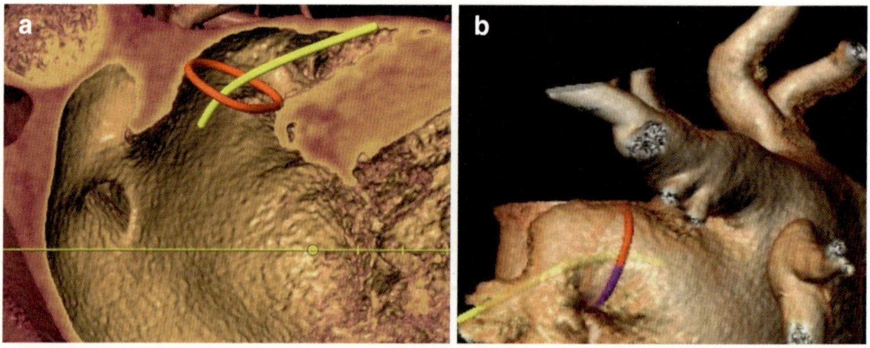

Fig. 5.5 Exemplary CT images of two patients illustrating the anatomic location of Watchman landing zone employed for correct sizing. (**a**, **b**) Internal and external imaging of a broccoli-type LAA. Watchman landing zone diameters are measured from the Cx ridge to a point approx. 1–2 cm distal to the coumadin ridge. Note the proximal ridge between the two lobes within the LAA. (**c**, **d**) Internal and external imaging of a classic chicken wing anatomy

Largest diameter LAA ostium mm	Watchman
16-18	21
18-20	24
21-23	27
24-26	30
27-30	33

Fig. 5.6 Sizing scheme of the Watchman device aiming for a compression of around 20% based on TEE measurements. Sizing is done by the largest diameter measured by TEE (mostly 135°) and/or angiography (RAO 15°, caudal 20°). The depth of the LAA is usually not easy to determine; measurement is therefore not required but is visualized by the Watchman sheath and its markers

- transseptal puncture inferior/posterior, heparin to ACT > 250sec
- exchange to Watchman double curve sheath with stiff wire in the left superior pulmonary vein
- 6F standard pigtail catheter to negotiate depth of LAA in a superior, anterior lobe; Watchman double curve follows
- visualize LAA by echo and angio, sizing
- delivery of Watchman device to LAA, careful air managment
- PASS-criteria
  - position proximal/distal/ideal?
  - anchoring correct? – tug test
  - sizing appropiate? –measure compression
  - sealing appropiate–test leakage next to device in all TEE view´s
- release of device
- close femoral access i.e. Proglide
- decide on post-procedural drug regimen:
  - warfarin 45 days followed by DPT to 6 months, then aspirin monotherapy
  - DAPT 3 months followed by aspirin monotherapy
  - NOAC therapy 3 months followed by aspirin monotherapy

Fig. 5.7 Watchman LAA closure: Step-by-step

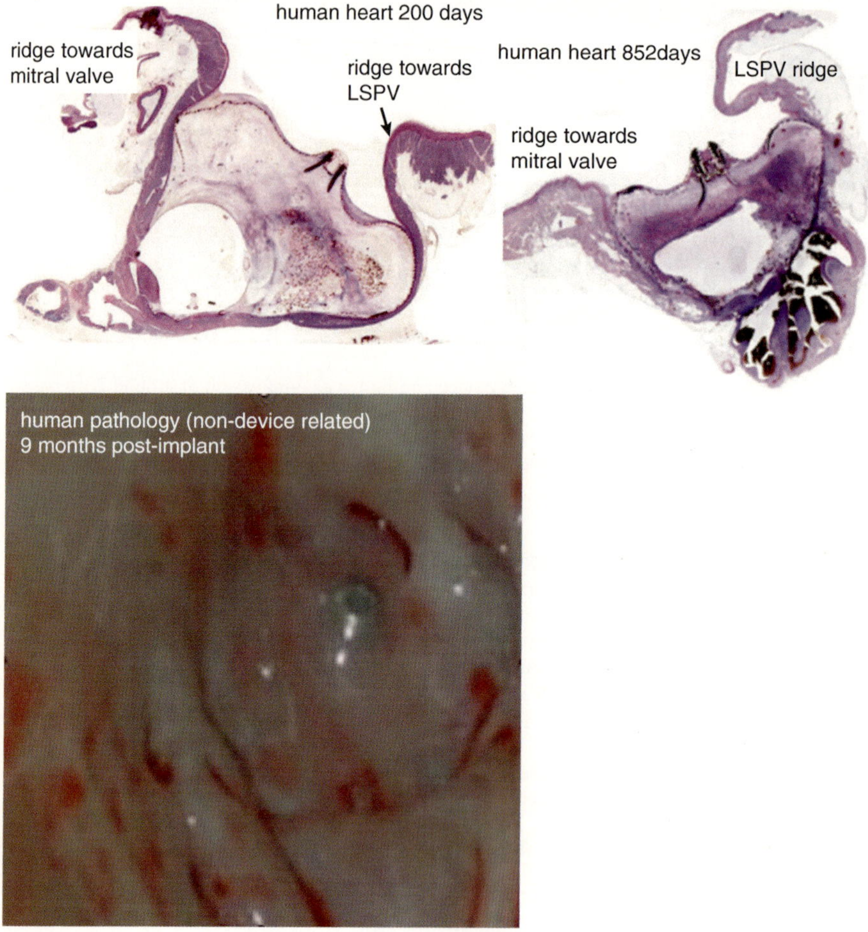

Fig. 5.8 Human histologic and pathologic analysis of implanted Watchman devices completely endothelialized and with organized tissue behind the fabric. Images courtesy of R. Virmani presented at EuroPCR 2013

is the most atraumatic strategy. The author prefers to perform this step in an LAO 40° angiographic angle as this allows to easily visualize the wire entering the LSPV (Fig. 5.10).

If the optimal position has been achieved through transseptal puncture, passing the wire through the SL1 sheath will automatically land in the LAA. A posterior movement (9 o'clock) is necessary to enter the LSPV after careful pullback of the SL1 sheath best guided by echo; this step has led the sheath to prolapse back into the right atrium or the sheath to be located below the ridge between LSPV and LAA. Some operators therefore favour to use a diagnostic multipurpose catheter together with a soft Terumo wire to negotiate the LSPV and exchange to a stiff wire

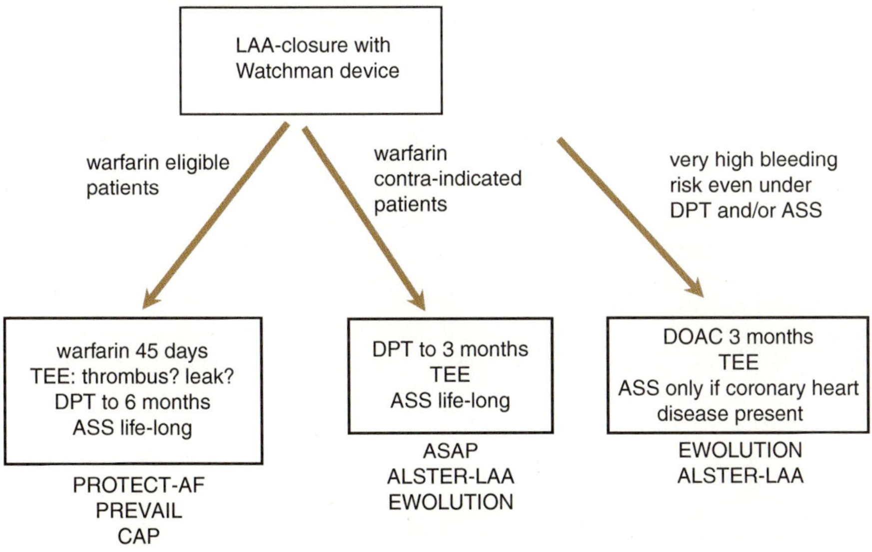

Fig. 5.9 Antithrombotic treatment options following LAA closure with the Watchman device. Studies supporting the various strategies are named below the options. In Europe most patients receive dual antiplatelet therapy for 3 months following LAA closure. US-based trials have included warfarin-eligible patients and have therefore used warfarin post-procedurally

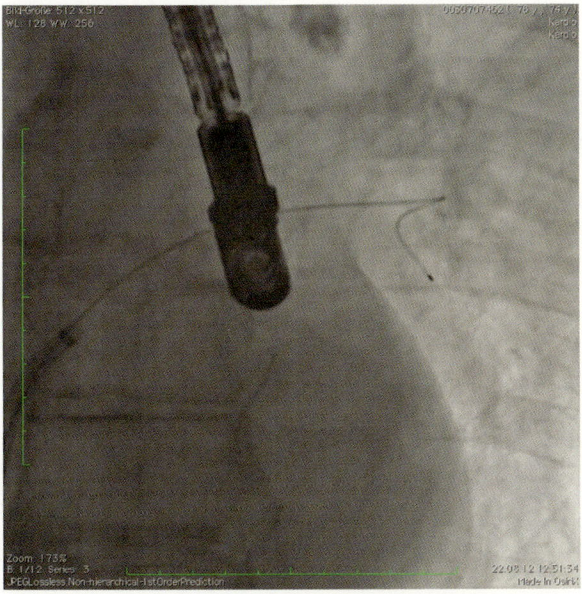

Fig. 5.10 Case example: following transseptal puncture, a stiff wire with a soft tip (i.e. Amplatzer superstiff 250 cm, Supracore 260 cm) is advanced into the superior pulmonary vein as seen in a LAO 40° angiographic view. The wire is clearly outside the epicardial border thus documenting the correct position in the LSPV. It is *not recommended* to exchange the sheath with the wire positioned in the LAA due to several perforations with life threatening pericardial effusions that occurred with this technique

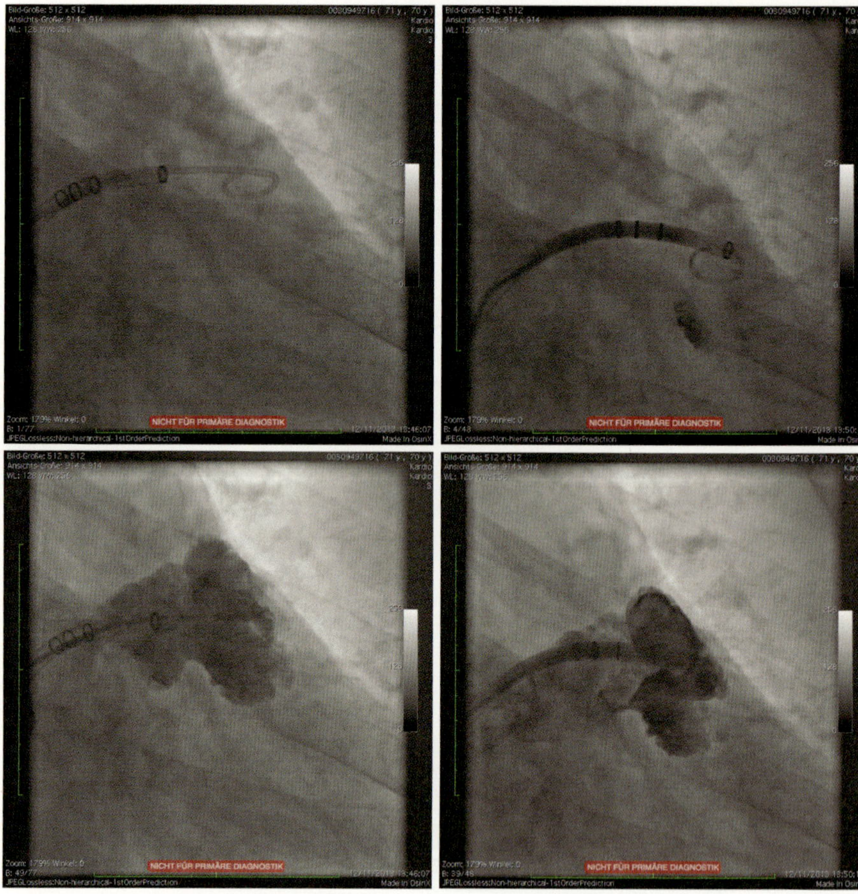

Fig. 5.11 Case example: after exchange to the Watchman sheath a 6F pigtail catheter is advanced into the LAA and used as a rail for atraumatic positioning of the sheath into the distal part of the LAA

over the MP catheter. Once the stiff wire has achieved a position deep in the LSPV outside the epicardial border, the Watchman sheath is advanced into the left atrium. Both the groin/pelvic area and the septum may pose some resistance that might lead the wire to prolapse back into the LA or even RA. Careful wire management is necessary to prevent this (Fig. 5.11).

It should be mentioned that from the moment of transseptal puncture air management becomes an important issue. Air embolism during sheath or wire exchange is a life threating complication. Preventive measures include the following:

– positive pressure in the LA prior to any manipulation best achieved by applying 1 l of saline soulution before the procedure and to monitor LA pressure; aim is >10 mmHg.

- sufficient LA pressure is also an important measure to correctly size the LAA ostium; some of the rare embolizations have occurred due to inaccurate sizing of the LAA in hypovolemia.
- stable sedation without the patient coughing and a guedel tube in place for airway management is mandatory. An episode of apnea will lead to negative pressure in the LA once it is resolved.

5.3 Sizing the LAA Watchman Landing Zone

Maximal diameter measurements to decide on device size are performed by 2D TEE at 0°, 45°, 90° and 135° approximately 1–2 cm from the ridge to the pulmonary vein at the superior border and the Cx traversing the inferior ridge. CT illustrates nicely the landing zone (Figs. 5.3, 5.4 and 5.5). Appropriate sizing allows the procedure to be finished with the first device chosen achieving complete clinical closure, defined as no or minimal (<5 mm) leakage in over 80% of patients. A sizing scheme currently used in many European centers is depicted in Fig. 5.6.

- Both TEE sizing as well as angiographic measurements to minimize underestimation of the landing zone are recommended (Figs. 5.12, 5.13, 5.14, 5.15 and 5.16)

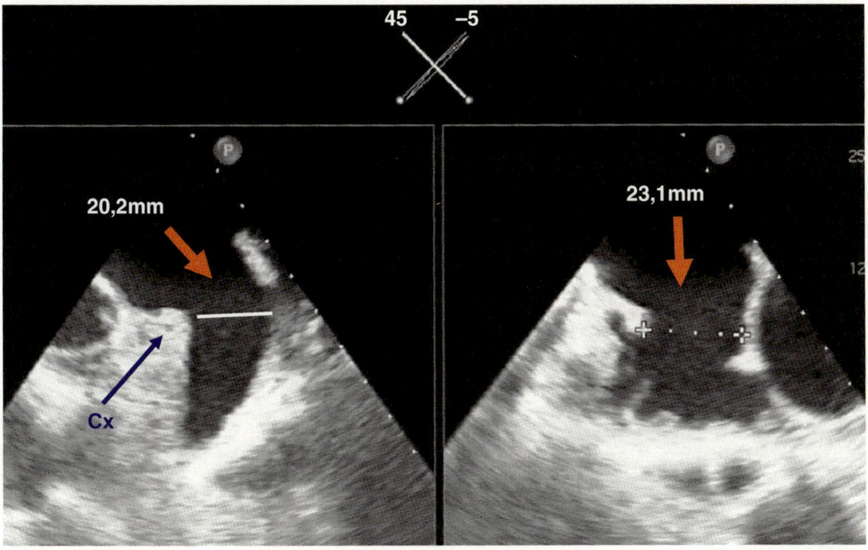

Fig. 5.12 Case example: exemplary orthogonal TEE measurements by X-plane 45°/130° of the LAA Watchman landing zone by TEE. The larger diameter is used for decision on Watchman device sizing according to the sizing scheme. The largest diameter is often found in the 135° view. According to the sizing scheme (see Fig. 6.6) this LAA should be closed with a 27 mm device

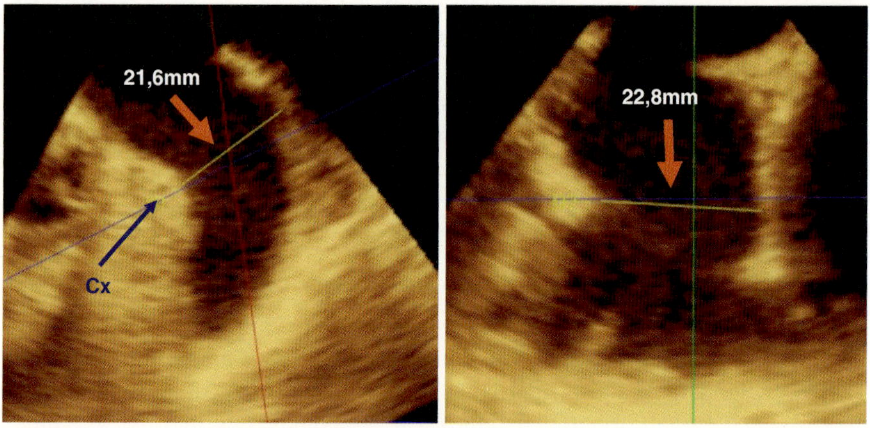

Fig. 5.13 Case example: exemplary orthogonal TEE measurements after 3D reconstruction of the LAA ostium by TEE. According the sizing scheme (see Fig. 6.6) this LAA should be closed with a 27 mm device

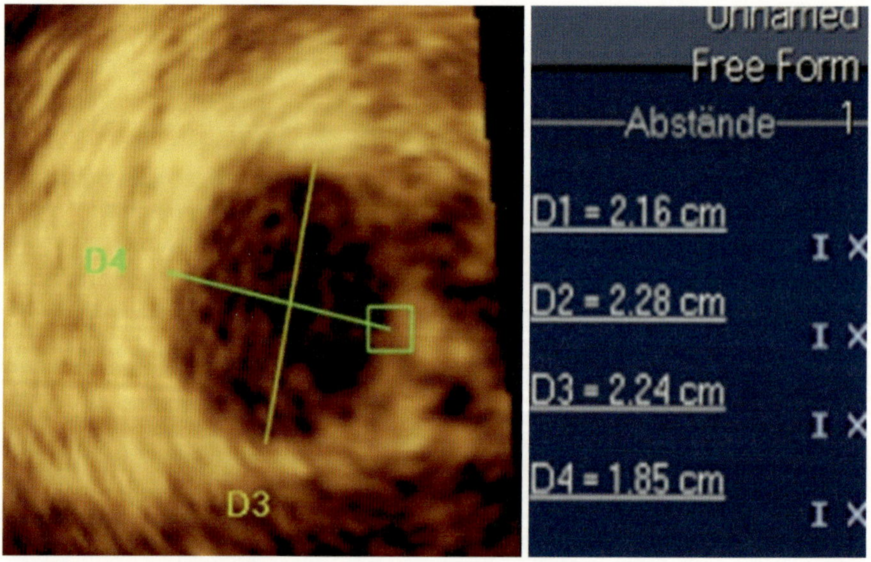

Fig. 5.14 Case example: alternative sizing by 3D reconstruction of the LAA ostium and measurement of largest diameter. According the sizing scheme (see Fig. 6.6) this LAA should be closed with a 27 mm device

- The largest diameter measured is used to decide which device size to choose.
- The largest diameter is found most often in the 135° view (Fig. 5.12 right panel). X-plane has proven to be helpful to visualize the Watchman landing zone
- 3D TEE reconstruction can visualize the oval orifice of the LAA and may be employed by those experienced in echo guidance of structural heart interventions structural heart echo guiding (Figs. 5.13 and 5.14)

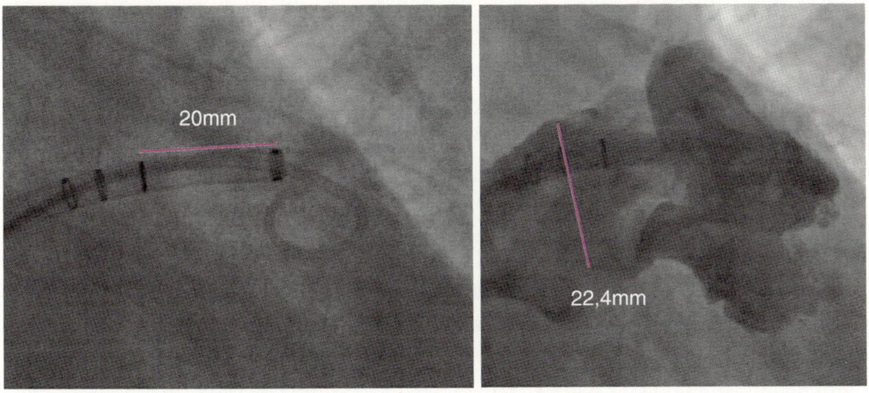

Fig. 5.15 Case example: angiographic sizing of the LAA ostium employing the Watchman sheath markers for normalization of the QCA program. According the sizing scheme (see Fig. 6.6) this LAA should be closed with a 27 mm device

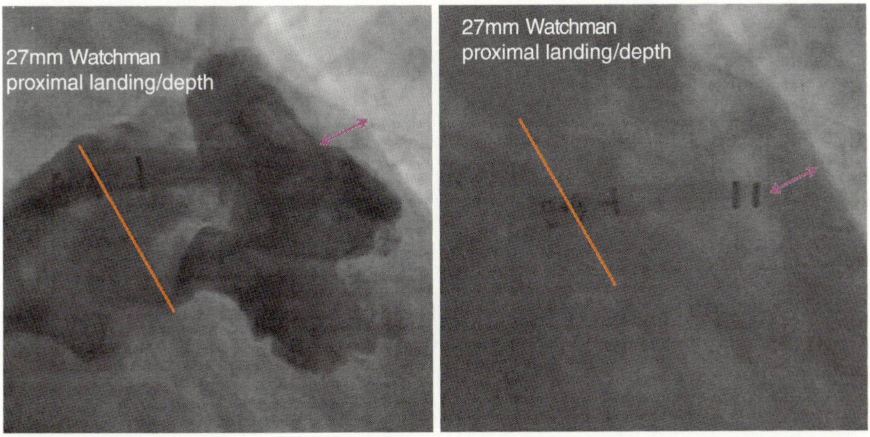

Fig. 5.16 Case example: after air-free exchange to the Watchman delivery system the distal point for device release is easily visualized by the distance to the epicardial border in an RAO caudal angiographic view. According the sizing scheme (see Fig. 6.6) this LAA should be closed with a 27 mm device—the sheath allows to estimate where the 27 mm proximal end will be localized

- Angiographic measurements are routine in many labs; the RAO caudal (RAO 20°, caudal 15°) view is often the default projection. Markers on the Watchman sheath may be used for normalization of the QCA settings (Fig. 5.15)
- As a rule of thumb, the device should be two sizes larger than the largest diameter measurement (Fig. 5.6)

Some centers, especially in France, Denmark and Italy, are regularly employing CT analysis prior to Watchman implantation for sizing (Figs. 5.4 and 5.5). Specialized CT analysis tools similar to TAVI workflows are available from 3MENSIO. Such measurements can also be performed by the DICOM reader OSIRIX MD. The measurements appear to be valid and allow for a straight forward workflow. Similar to the evolving TAVI workflow CT might allow to avoid periprocedural TEE in experienced hands where transseptal puncture and exclusion of peri-device leakage can possibly be guided by angiography.

5.4 Watchman Implantation Step-by-Step

Once the Watchman sheath is located in the left atrium, a standard 6F pigtail catheter is advanced into the LA and used to atraumatically negotiate the LAA. This is best achieved in a RAO caudal projection. As a default strategy, the pigtail should be placed in the most superior/anterior or middle lobe (broccoli type LAA) or even in the depth of a chicken wing LAA (Fig. 5.11). As long as only the pigtail but not a wire is used to probe the LAA the risk of pericardial effusion is minimal. For advancing the Watchman sheath to the depth of the LAA the pigtail may be stabilized internally with a standard J-wire.

- final landing zone diameter measurements are taken with contrast injected into the LAA over the pigtail catheter in an RAO caudal projection.
- using an ACIST system a setting of 7 ml/min flow and 15 ml total volume provides good visualization of the LAA.
- the device should be prepared prior to removing the pigtail from the Watchman sheath
- no distal movement of the sheath should occur after this step to prevent pericardial effusion

Preparation of the device:

- the Watchman device needs to be checked for correct connection of the delivery cable and the device by moving the device back in the sheath.
- the Watchman device is flushed so that no air remains in the system.

Only after these steps have been performed, the pigtail is removed from the Watchman sheath and exchanged for the device. Prior to the device leaving the distal end of the sheath any air in the sheath should be removed either by constant flush or by a backbleeding.

- the device is advanced until only 5 mm are left before the device connects to the port of the sheath. At this point, the radiopaque markers at the distal end of the device and the sheath align.
- the final connection is made by pulling the sheath back (Fig. 5.16).
- release of the nitinol device is performed by pulling back the device delivery system together with the sheath now firmly attached to each other.
- the device should be kept stable at a distal position; the pericardial edge may serve as a landmark in the RAO caudal projection (Fig. 5.16). This may require some push on the device as the sheath straightens when moving back.

If the device does not fulfill the release criteria (see below), the device may be partially recaptured and released at a more proximal position. For more distal release a full recapture and repositioning of the sheath with a pigtail is recommended. This technique may be modified with growing experience of the implanters, yet it will possibly increase the risk of pericardial effusion. Therefore starting device release at the most distal position achievable in the first place is recommended as the default strategy.

5.5 Release Criteria

Four criteria (PASS) must be fulfilled prior to device release:

- *P*osition of the device, including LA protrusion, is checked by angiography and echo. Less than half the depth of the device should protrude in the LA in order to secure the PET fabric to prevent any thrombi from leaving the LAA (see device features).
- A tug test confirms *A*nchoring; device position should be checked again afterwards. No change of device position should be observed. (Fig. 5.17). If necessary, the maneuver is repeated until there is clearly no movement of the device position in relation to the LAA.
- *S*eal: Successful closure of all lobes of the LAA must be documented in all four TEE projections (0°, 45°, 90°, 135°) again using X-plane if available (Fig. 5.18). A colour jet >5 mm at the LAA ostium previously employed for measurement should not be accepted. If device sizing was correct leakage is most often solved by a partial recapture and a more proximal release of the device possibly accepting a "shoulder" protruding into the LA.
- *S*ize: compression of the device at the most proximal position with surrounding tissue is measured and should document compression of the device of around 20% (Fig. 5.19).

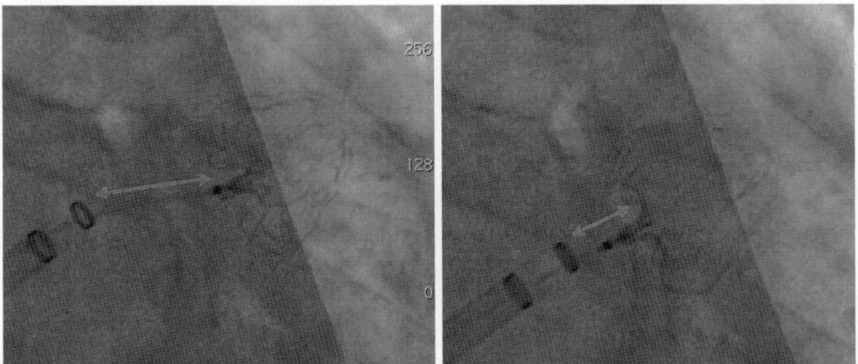

Fig. 5.17 Case example: the device shows a typical strawberry configuration after successful release. A *tug test* is performed by pulling the connector wire to confirm anchoring. The device should be stable both by angiographic and TEE criteria

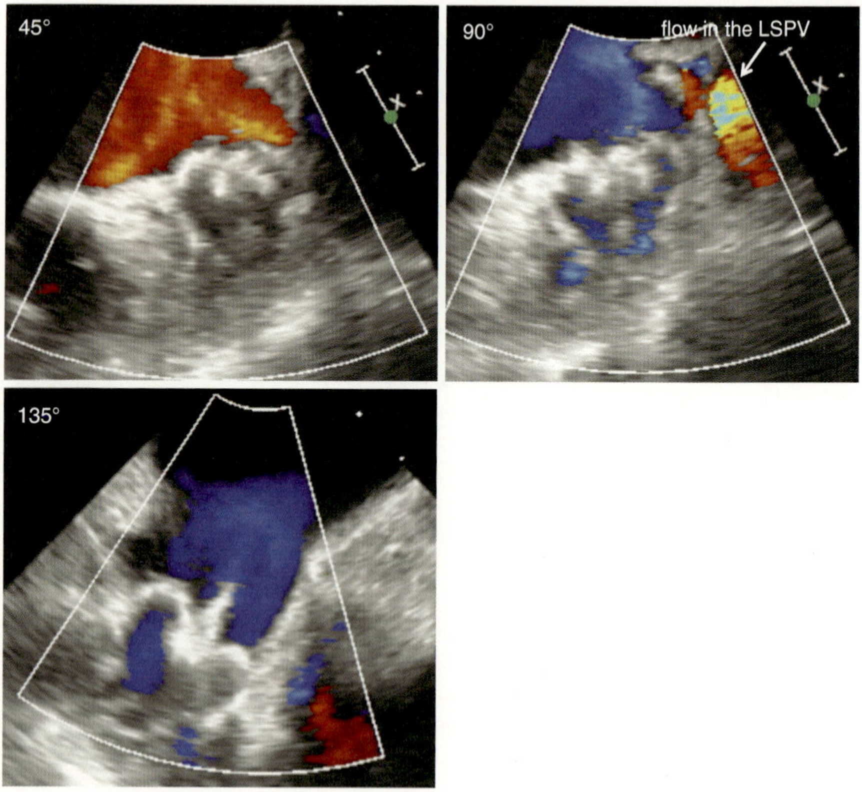

Fig. 5.18 Case example: echocardiographic assessment of *leakage* next to the device. Any peridevice leakage less than 5 mm is acceptable as no increased clinical event rate is reported (V. Reddy et al.; PROTECT AF subgroup analysis)

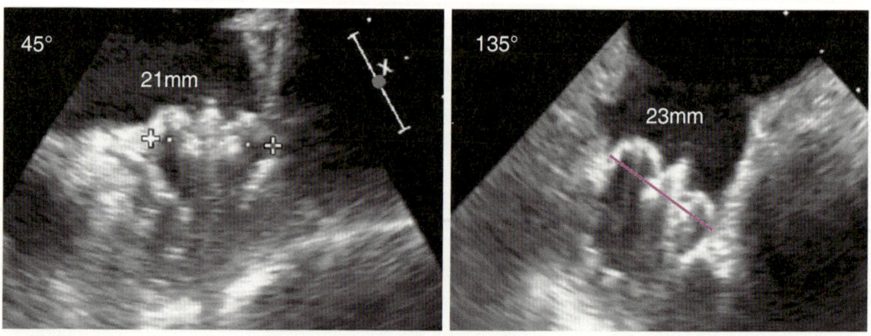

Fig. 5.19 Case example: assessment of *compression and position* at the LAA Watchman landing zone is performed in all four TEE views (0°, 45°, 90° and 135°). Device compression should be around 20%. Measurement is performed at the most proximal position of the device where the LAA diameter was previously measured

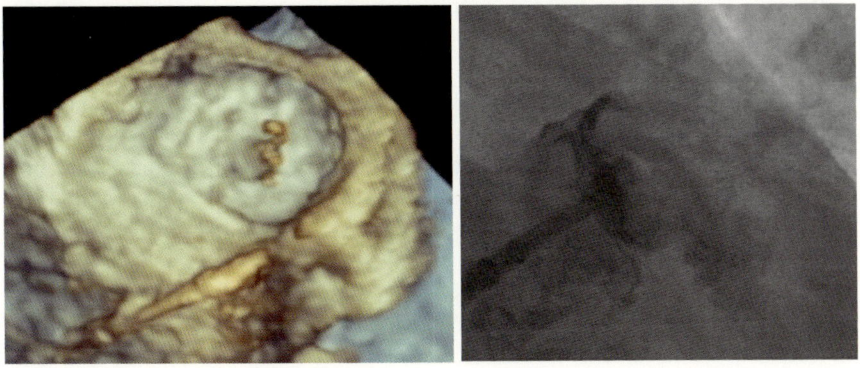

Fig. 5.20 Case example: final position of the device in 3D TEE and angiographic visualization

The four release criteria can be memorized by the acronym "PASS" standing for position, anchoring, sealing and size (=compression) (Fig. 5.20). Following confirmation of LAA sealing and stable position of the device, the delivery cable is turned counter-clockwise until the device is released. A final check is performed prior to removing the sheath from the left atrium. Afterwards, a potential tear in the septum that could lead to a larger ASD is evaluated by TEE. This complication is a rare event. Larger TEE series performed in the context of pulmonary vein isolation have showed that smaller defects heal over a time course of 6 to 12 months.

5.6 Sheath Removal and Hemostasis

Groin hematoma is a common complication after the use of the 14F outer diameter Watchman sheath. A Z-stitch is commonly used to achieve hemostasis—it needs to be removed the next day. Further, the Proglide occluder system is in regular use by several centers, also in the venous system. Another device commonly used in this context is the FemoStop. Of note, the FemoStop needs to be removed to prevent complete hemostasis in the venous femoral system as thrombus formation leading to pulmonary emboli have occurred.

5.7 Post-Procedural Care and Drug Regimen

After LAA occlusion a patient is usually monitored for one night in order to detect early complications like pericardial effusion. The standard program includes:

- Transthoracic echo (TTE) to exclude pericardial effusion
- TTE to exclude device embolization. If a device embolizes it is often found in the descending aorta (see Chapter 9).

If none of the above mentioned complications have occurred, the patient can usually be discharged the day after the procedure.

The fabric of the device immediately prevents any thrombi from leaving the LAA. The device endothelializes over 3–6 months (Fig. 5.8). As thrombus at the LA facing side of the device may occur, transient post-procedural anticoagulation might be necessary (Fig. 5.9). Post-implantation drug regimens for Watchman implantation were initially standardized to 45 days of warfarin followed by dual antiplatelet therapy to 6 months. At this time complete endothelialization is achieved and drug therapy could be switched to aspirin monotherapy in the randomized US trials PROTECT-AF and PREVAIL and the continued access protocol ("CAP") registry. In Europe implanters have mostly treated patients with a relative or absolute contraindication to warfarin. This has led to most patients being treated with dual antiplatelet therapy directly after the procedure; this strategy was found to be safe and effective in several smaller series (ASAP, ALSTER-LAA registry) and the large, prospective EWOLUTION registry. No increased risk of thrombus at the device or post-procedural stroke in the first three months after the procedure were observed (see Chap. 2.3). This strategy can therefore be regarded as safe and effective for patients who are not able to take warfarin even for a short period of 45 days. EWOLUTION has also demonstrated that other post-procedural drug regimens may be feasible although with smaller patient numbers, namely no therapy at all, a single antiplatelet therapy and -most interestingly- NOAC therapy for 3 months post-implantation (Fig. 5.9). The latter came with the lowest event rate of all drug regimens regarding bleeding, and with rates of stroke and device-related thrombus comparable to warfarin therapy (see Chap. 2). In comparison to the current standard in Europe, namely dual antiplatelet therapy, it also carries the advantage of a short half life and in case of dabigatran the availability of a specific and highly effective antidote (idaruzimab). In patients with a very high risk of bleeding, post-procedural NOAC therapy, possibly even in reduced doses (i.e. 75 mg dabigatran BID), might therefore be the best available strategy. Further data are necessary to support this conclusion.

Acknowledgment The authors would like to thank Mrs. Elisa Vireca, MS, Boston Scientific, Diegem, Belgium for critical reading and helpful comments.

Chapter 6
Practical Watchman Implantation: Case Examples

6.1 Case Examples for the Watchman LAA Occluder

6.1.1 Shallow LAA: Watchman Implantation with "Shoulder" (Case 1)

Learning objective: standard technique for dual lobe LAA occlusion with limited depth.

If LAA depth is an issue as depicted in Case 1 (Figs. 6.1, 6.2, 6.3, 6.4, 6.5, 6.6, 6.7, 6.8, 6.9 and 6.10), the following technique is recommended:

- The landing zone is measured angiographically to be 17.6 mm (Fig. 6.1).
- Orthogonal measurement (Fig. 6.2) in X-plane by echo reveals a maximum diameter of 19.9 mm at 45°; the 135° angle corresponding to the RAO caudal angio measurement also measures 17.3 mm.
- 3D reconstruction of the LAA confirms an oval shape of 19 × 15 mm (Figs. 6.3 and 6.4). The maximum diameter of 19 mm suggests a device size of 24 mm.
- Following deep insertion of the watchman sheath over the pigtail "rail" into the depth of the LAA (Fig. 6.1), the device is released by unsheathing the nitinol frame. Immediately after release a tug test is performed (Fig. 6.5).
- Echo and angiography show that angiographic visualization finds the device partially protrudes to partially protrude into the left atrium (Figs. 6.6 and 6.8). No peridevice leakage is observed (Fig. 6.7). The maximum shoulder depth is only 9 mm (Fig. 6.8); this results in a complete seal of the LAA since 50% of the device equalling 12 mm is covered with fabric (Fig. 6.9). Final echo and angiographic images confirm the good result (Fig. 6.10).

M.W. Bergmann et al., *Clinical Cases in LAA Occlusion*,
DOI 10.1007/978-3-319-51431-4_6

RAO 30°, caudal 15°

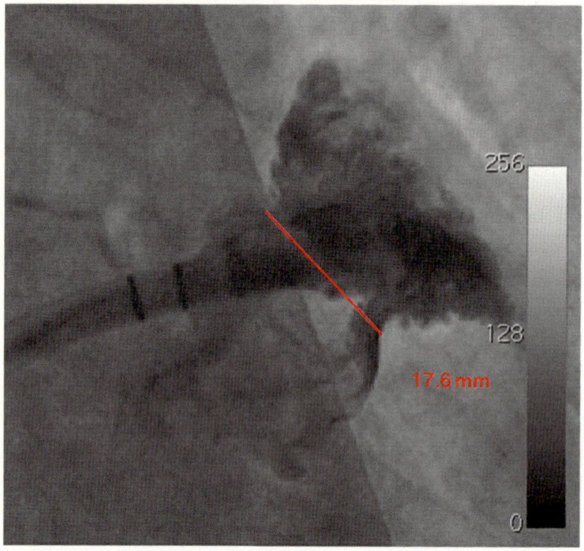

Fig. 6.1 Case 1: sizing of the LAA Watchman landing zone by angiography. The challenge in this particular case is that depth appears not to be sufficient at first glance. This measurement would suggest a 21 mm Watchman according to the sizing scheme, yet it might not be the largest diameter measured

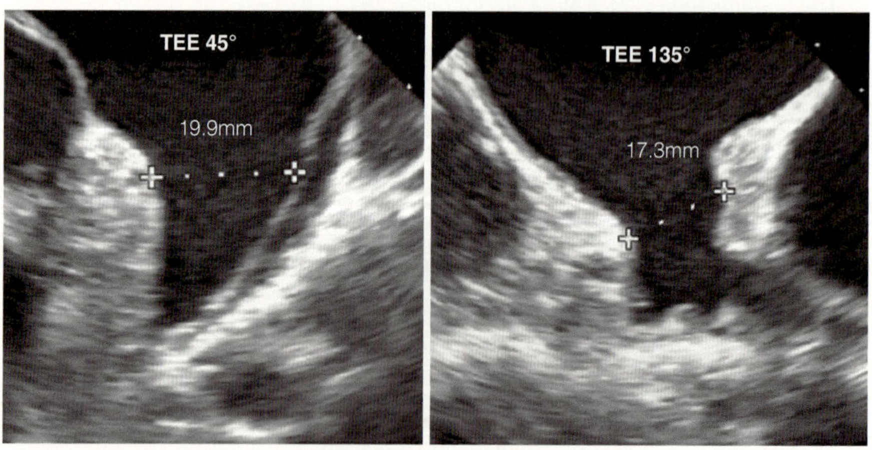

Fig. 6.2 Case 1: sizing of the LAA ostium by 2D echo/X-plane. This particular LAA has the largest diameter measured in 45° suggesting a 24 mm Watchman device to be the device of choice

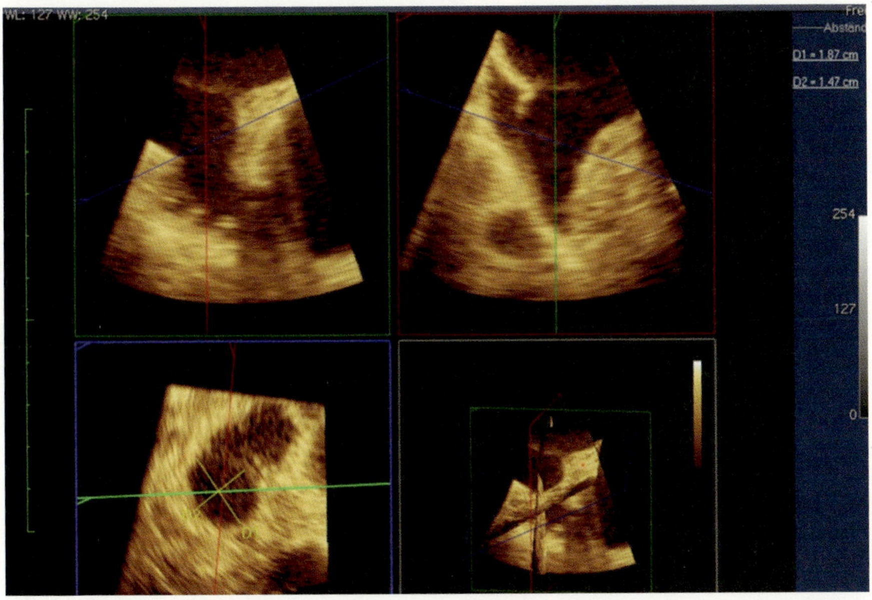

Fig. 6.3 Case 1: sizing of the LAA ostium by 3D echo employing Q-lab software for reconstruction; again a 24 mm Watchman device is recommended

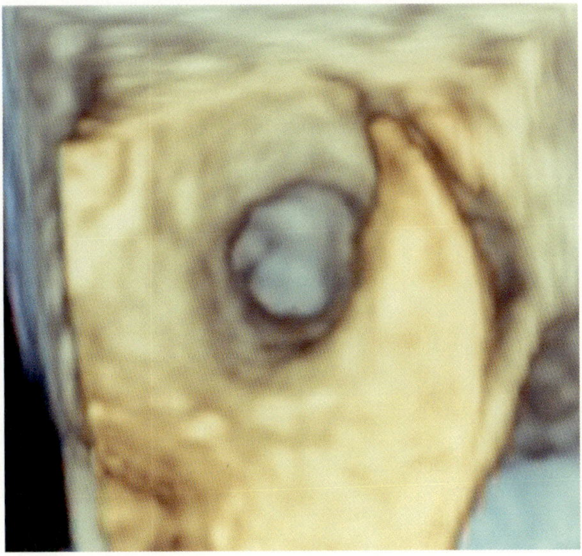

Fig. 6.4 Case 1: 3D reconstruction of the LAA

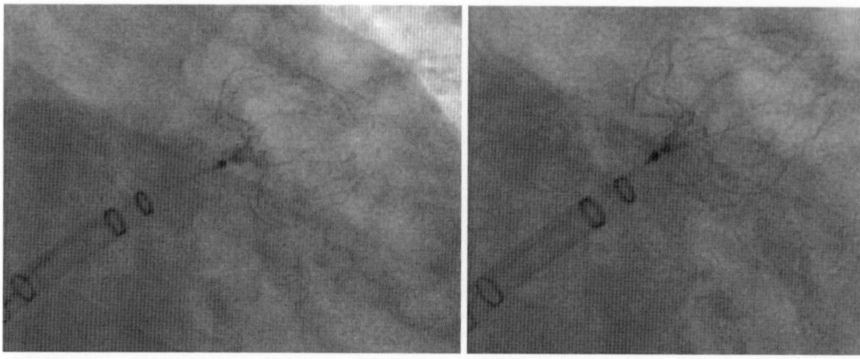

Fig. 6.5 Case 1: tug test directly after release; Watchman has taken the typical configuration and unfolded completely. Note that the distal part is compressed to about 50% width compared to the proximal part

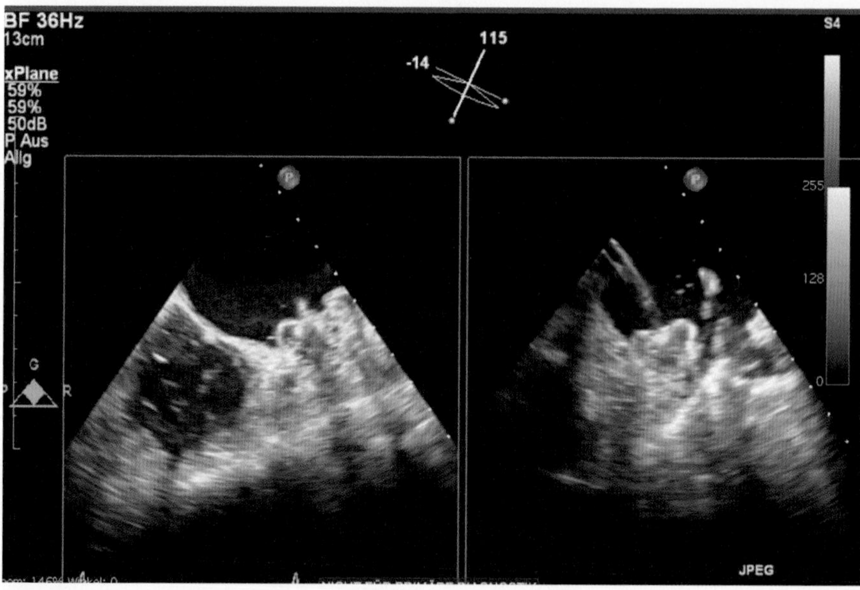

Fig. 6.6 Case 1: 24 mm Watchman device after release. Note that the depth measured underestimate the true landing zone

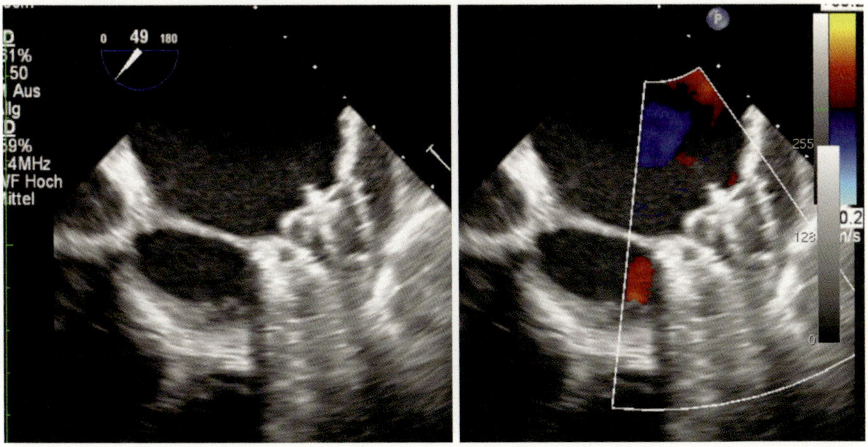

Fig. 6.7 Case 1: no leakage around device is detected. All release criteria (position, anchoring (tug test), size and sealing) are fulfilled

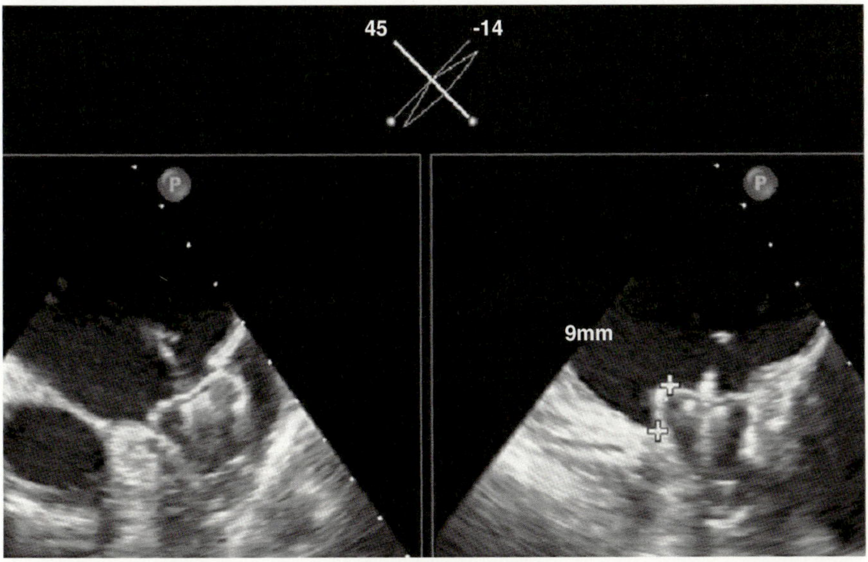

Fig. 6.8 Case 1: position assessment: a protrusion to the left atrium ("shoulder") is observed. If this protrusion measures less than 50% of the diameter (Watchman 24 mm: 12 mm) in any of the four TEE views (0°, 45°, 90°, 135°), position can be accepted as the device still covers the LAA with PET fabric preventing thrombi from exiting the LAA

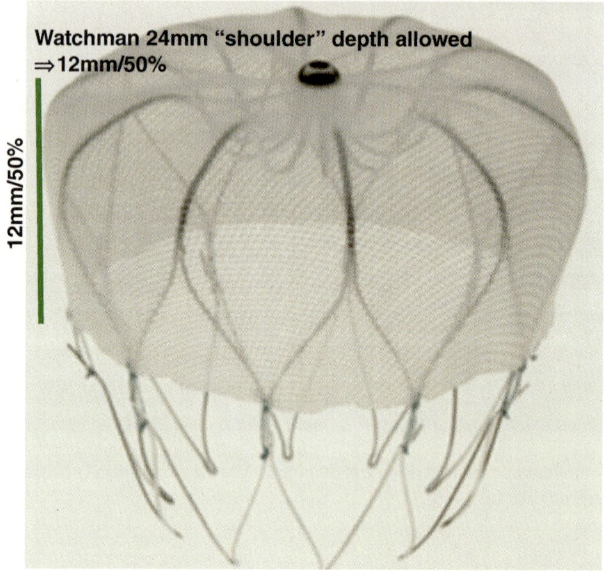

Fig. 6.9 Watchman device: the fabric covers 50% of the height of the device; a shoulder of around 12 mm can be accepted for a 24 mm device

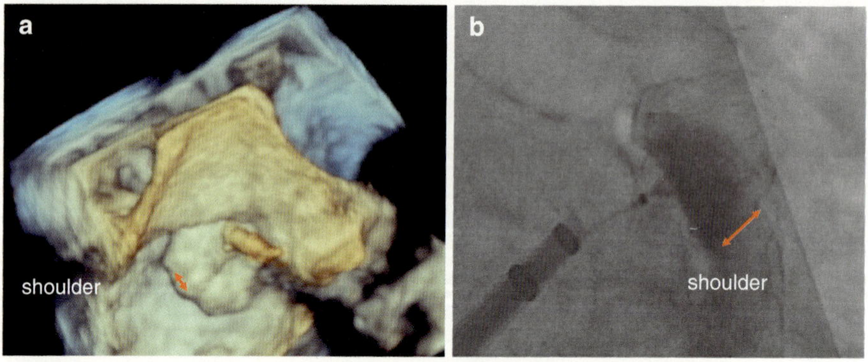

Fig. 6.10 Case 1: final position as visualized by 3D echo (**a**) and angiography (**b**)

6.1.2 Dual Lobe LAA (Case 2)

Learning objective: standard technique if the anchoring lobe is limiting device expansion due to a proximal interlobar ridge.

A common challenge is to close a LAA with two lobes connected by a ridge that is protruding proximally. For successful closure of this anatomy the following strategy is recommended:

- landing zone measurements find 23 mm to be the largest diameter, this time in 45° (Fig. 6.11)
- probing of the LAA with the pigtail demonstrate two large lobes with a proximal ridge (Fig. 6.12)

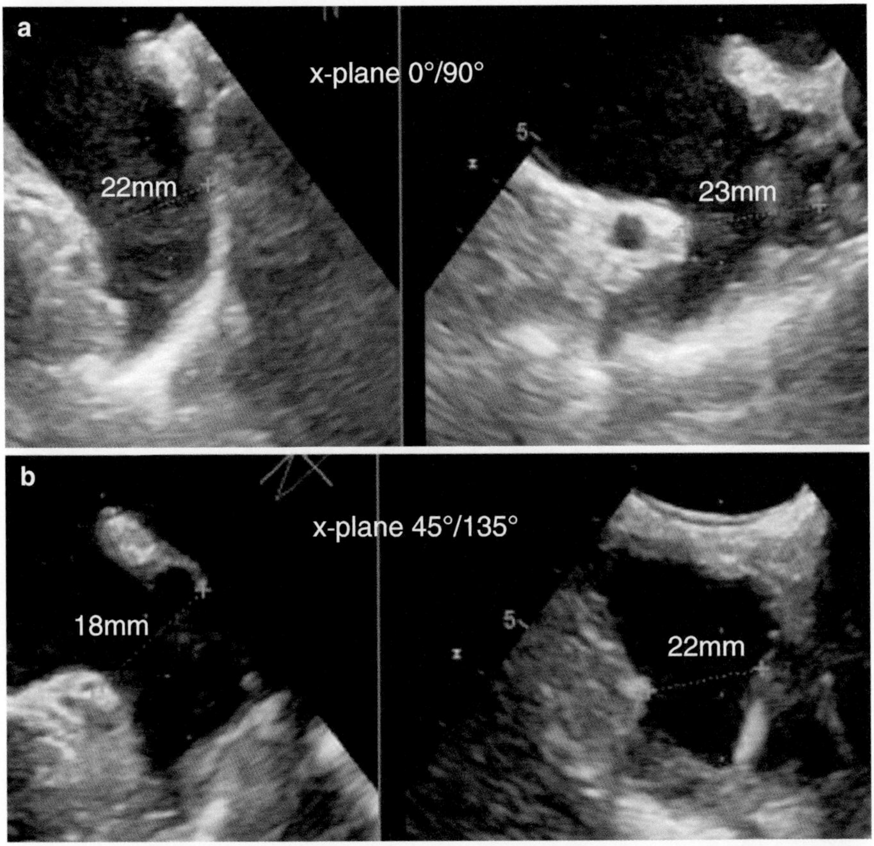

Fig. 6.11 Case 2: closure of a dual lobe LAA. (**a** + **b**) Echo measurements of the Watchman landing zone in all four planes employing the X-plane mode. The largest diameter is measured at 23 mm resulting in a device size of 27 mm

- the 27 mm Watchman is released from the superior lobe; if a first distal release doesn't cover the inferior lobe the device must be positioned more proximal (Figs. 6.13 and 6.14)
- only gaps <5 mm are allowed, measured at the smallest entry with colour flow next to the device (Fig. 6.14b)
- 3D imaging confirms successful closure of this particular LAA (Fig. 6.15)

6.1.3 LAA with Inferior Take-off (Case 3)

Learning objective: a LAA with inferior direction requires specific measures to limit device protrusion into the left atrium.

If the LAA takes an inferior direction some challenges might occur to position the Watchman without a shoulder. The following technique is recommended:

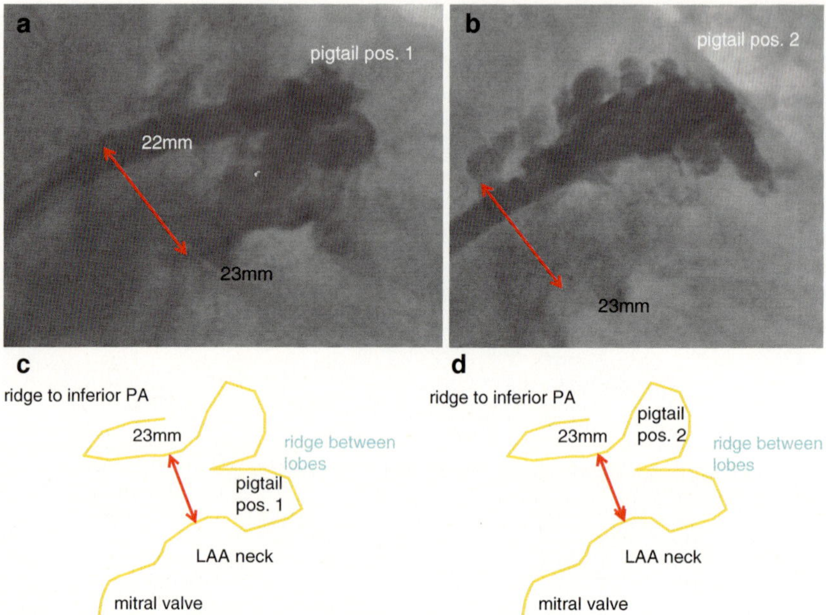

Fig. 6.12 Case 2: closure of a dual lobe LAA. (**a** + **c**) pigtail in inferior lobe (position 1), (**b** + **d**) pigtail in superior lobe (position 2), the position to start Watchman release. In the RAO caudal angiographic projection the Watchman landing zone is measured to be 23 mm

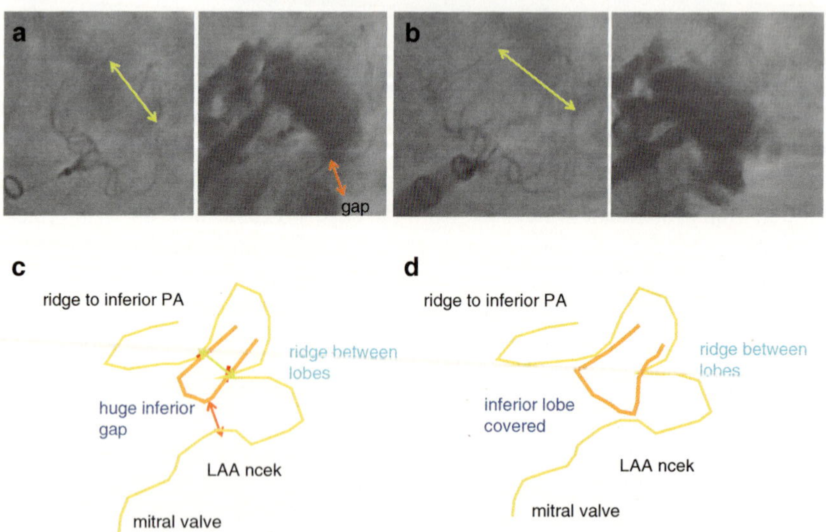

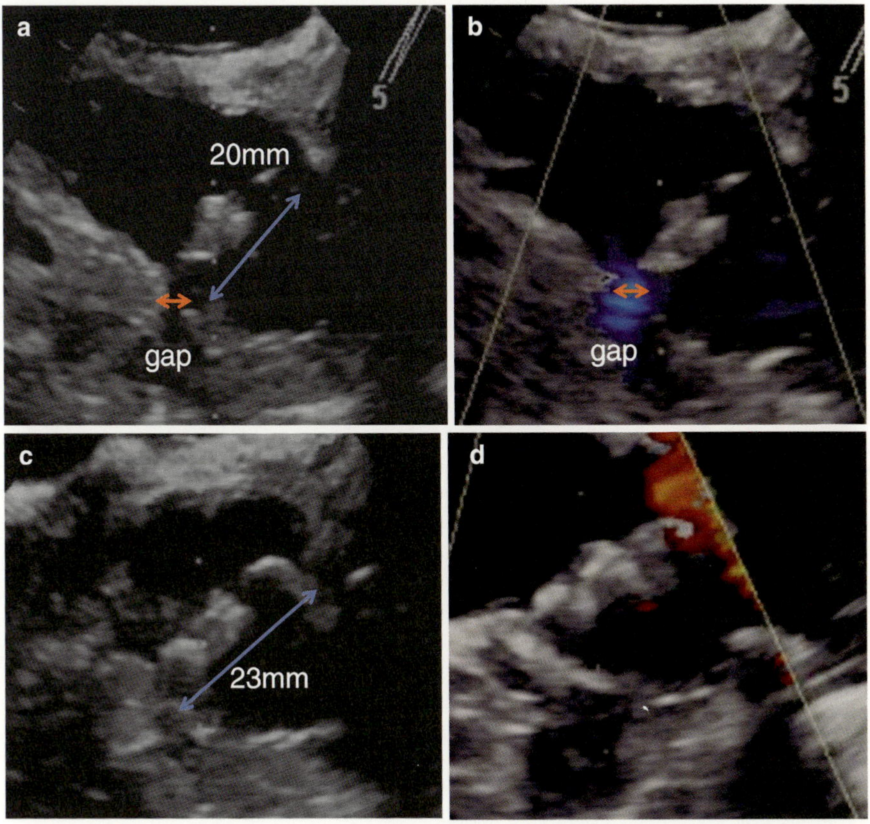

Fig. 6.14 Case 2: corresponding echo images to Fig. 6.33: The first release of a 27 mm Watchman (**a**, **b**) leaves a gap. The 27 mm device expands to only 20 mm; the explanation is found when looking at the angiographic images in 6.34: the interlobar ridge prevents the device to expand if released at this position. Now the device is partially recaptured and released a few mm more proximal. This allows the proximal part of this 27 mm Watchman device to expand completely and cover the inferior lobe (**c**, **d**)

Fig. 6.13 Case 2: default strategy to close a multi-lobe LAA with the Watchman device. The first release of a 27 mm Watchman (**a**, **c**) leaves an inferior gap since the proximal ridge between the lobes prevents the device from covering the inferior lobe. Note the very high compression of the distal part of the device in that small superior lobe (*yellow arrow* **a** and **c**, see Fig. 6.32a). Now the device is partially recaptured and released a few mm more proximal. This allows the proximal part of the same Watchman device as in a/c to expand completely and to cover the inferior lobe (**b**, **d**)

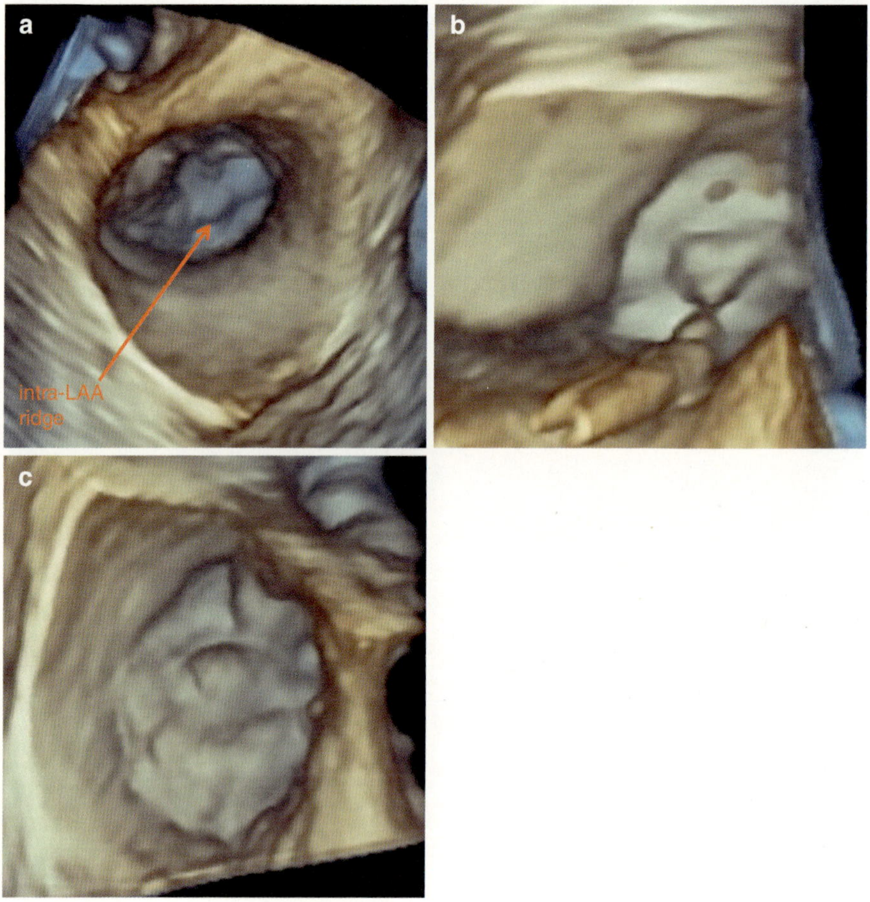

Fig. 6.15 Case 2: corresponding 3D Echo images to the images in Fig. 6.33 and 6.34: (**a**) Visualization of the the proximal ridge between the lobes to cover. (**b**) The first release of a 27 mm Watchman is very deep into the LAA. (**c**) The more proximal final position with a small protrusion into the LA (shoulder) completely covers the entrance to the LAA

- measure landing zone both in angio and echo; be aware that the proximal marker of the sheath orients to where a 33 mm device might land outside the LAA (Fig. 6.15 a and b)
- During release of the device from the distal LAA, a slight push is applied once 50% of the device is released. This enables the device to land exactly at the predefined landing zone (Fig. 6.16)
- checking sealing and anchoring by the PASS criteria suggest the device to be successfully deployed (Fig. 6.17)

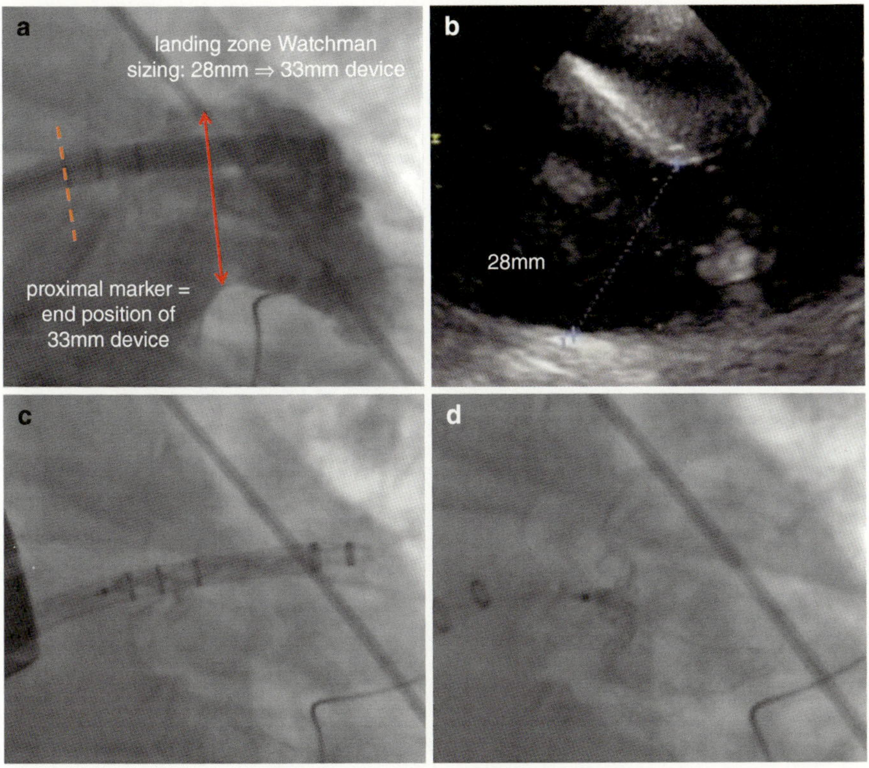

Fig. 6.16 Case 3: LAA morphology in an RAO caudal projection depicts an inferior take-off (**a**). Echo imaging does not provide information about the depth of the LAA but measures the Watchman landing zone also with 28 mm (**b**). "2-sizes up" leads to the decision of a 33 mm device w/o an issue of depth although the markers on the sheath suggest the device to protrude into the left atrium (**a**, *orange dotted line*). Release starts at the very distal end of the LAA (**c**). After release, the device shows its typical appearance(**d**)

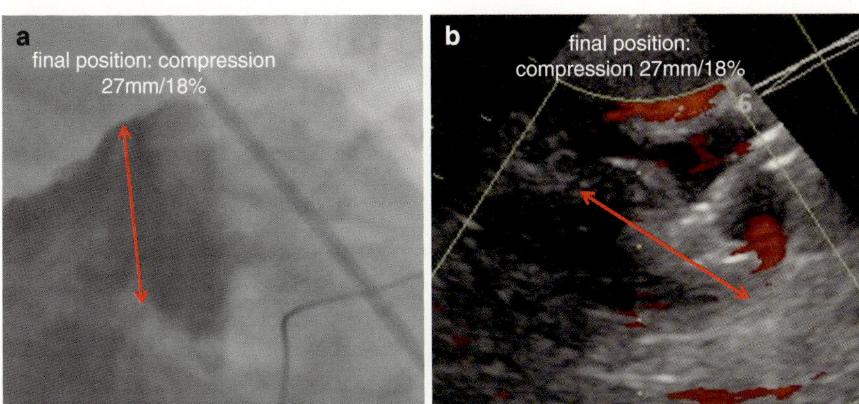

Fig. 6.17 Case 3: both angiographic (**a**) as well as echocardiographic images (**b**) confirm complete sealing of the LAA with a compression of the 33 mm device to 27 mm (6 mm/18%)

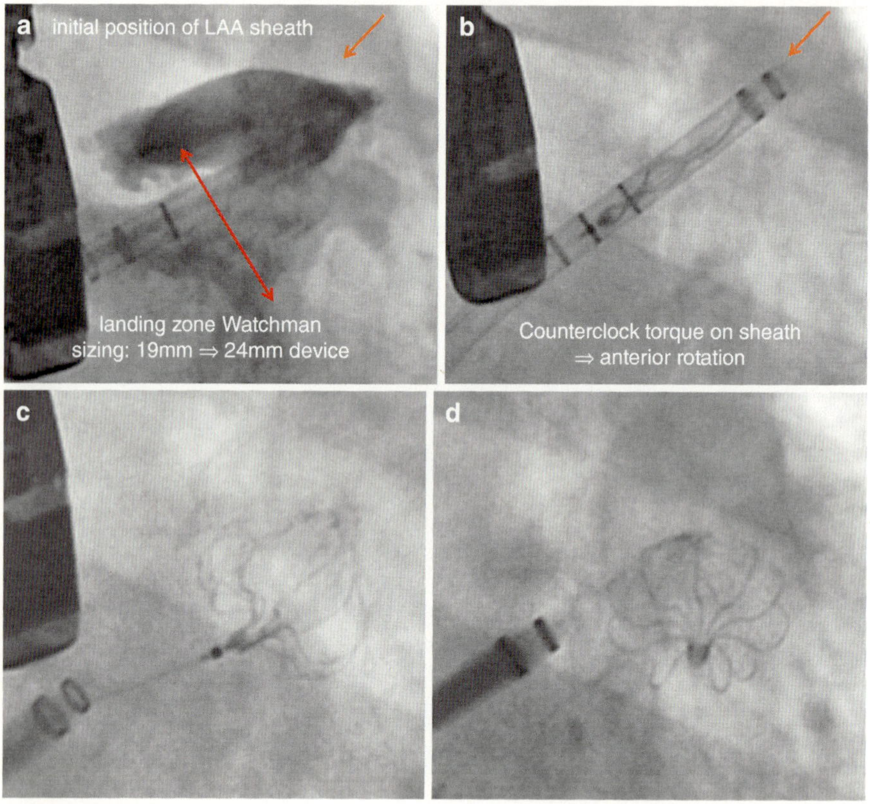

Fig. 6.18 Case 4: classical chicken wing morphology. Sufficient depth for device implantation is questionable. (**a**) The Pigtail catheter can be moved into the distal part of the LAA. (**b**) The sheath is positioned as distal as possible. (**c**) The 24 mm Watchman device is released from the sheath; if neccessary a slight push can be applied after 50% of the device is released from the delivery system (**d**) After testing the PASS-criteria, the device is released. In this case, the device orientates itself superiorly

6.1.4 LAA with Chicken Wing Morphology (Case 4)

Learning objective: chicken wing morphology requires special attention to position the sheath prior to device release.

In several patients, the LAA is turning 180° upwards shortly after the proximal Watchman landing zone. The following technique is recommended:

- Usually the pigtail can easily be placed into the distal part of the LAA despite the 180° turn. A standard 0.035 J-wire may help to stabilize the 6F pigtail when the Watchman double curve sheath is advanced as far as possible (Fig. 6.18b)
- during device release a constant counterclockwise torque on the sheath allows for a distal release of the 24 mm Watchman device

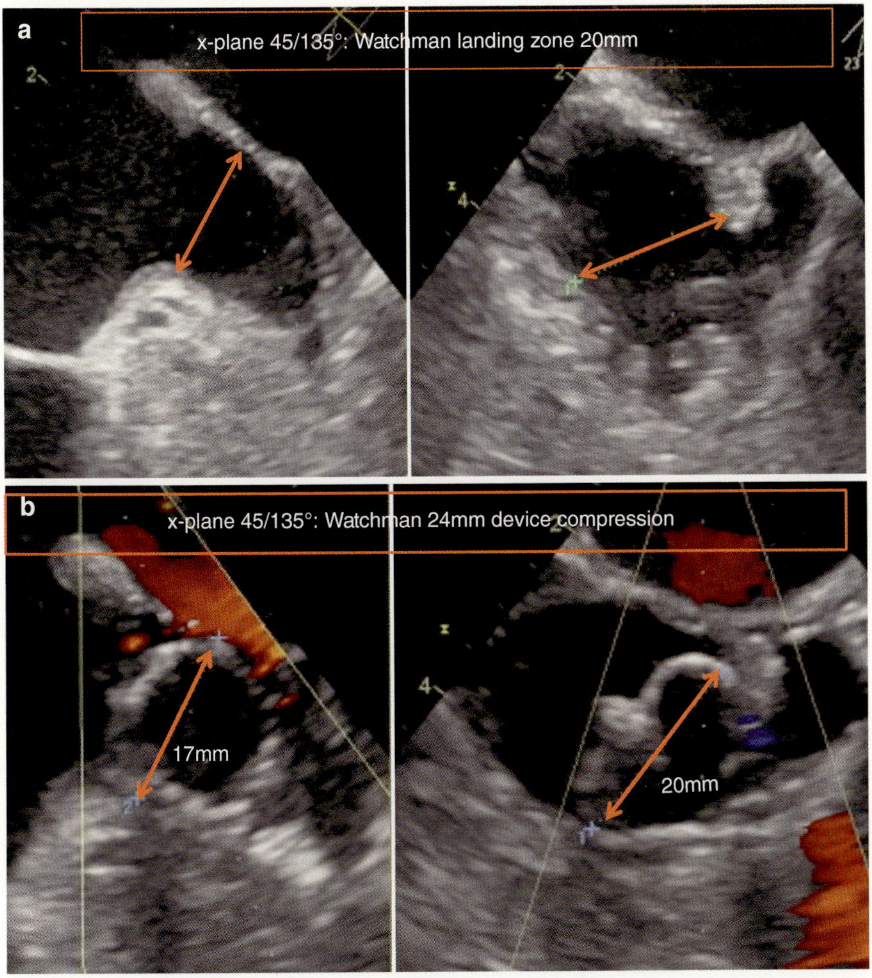

Fig. 6.19 Case 4: classical chicken wing morphology: (**a**) The chicken wing morphology is nicely visible; (**b**) successful closure of both the proximal part as well as the distal part of the LAA

- in this particular case the device orientates itself along the LAA axis after release
- successful closure is documented by angiography and echo (Figs. 6.19 and 6.20)

6.1.5 LAA with Dual Lobe Anatomy (Case 5)

Learning objective: LAA depth anatomy is difficult to understand and visualize. In case the device unfolds in an unexpected conformation, lobular structure and ridges are usually responsible.

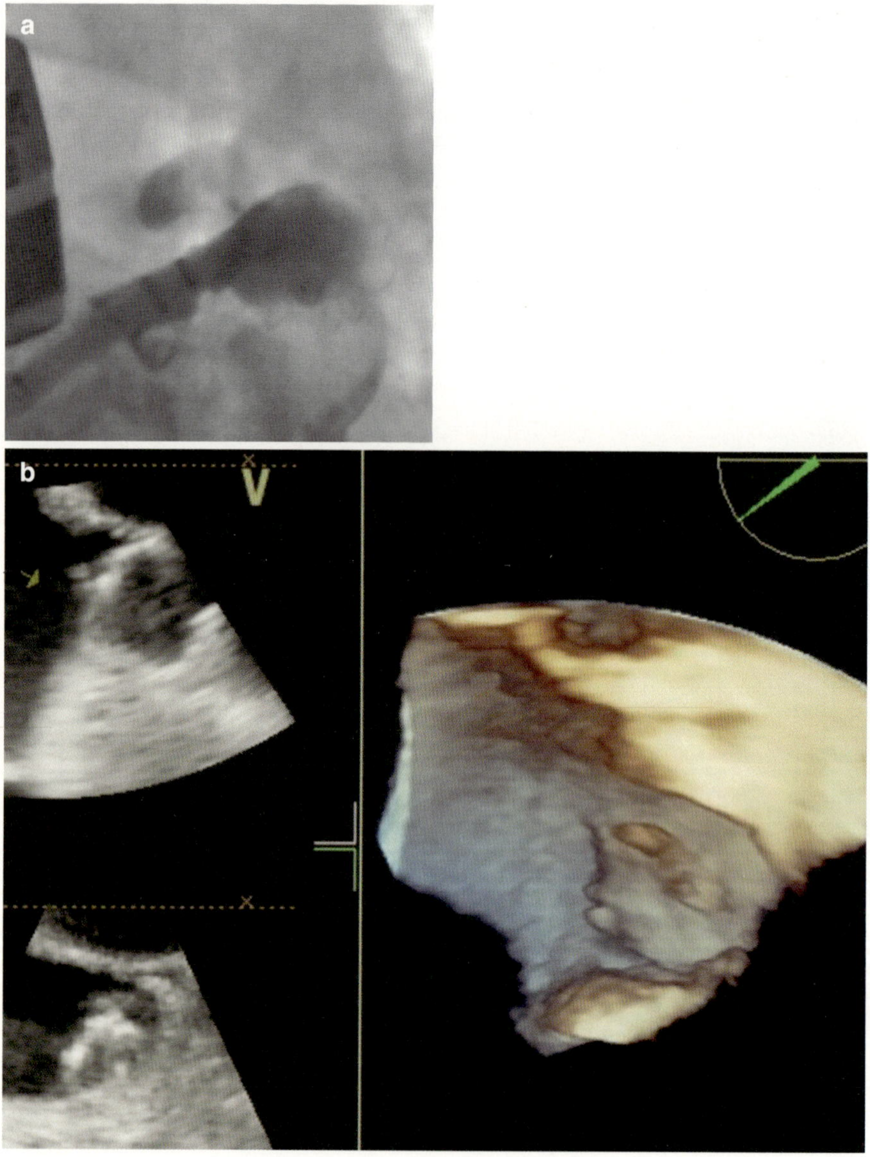

Fig. 6.20 Case 4: successful closure of a chicken wing morphology as judged by Angio (**a**) and echo (**b**) imaging

As shown above, dual lobe LAA with a proximal interlobar ridge is a common finding. The following technique is recommended:

- visualization of the LAA depth by angiography over pigtail to understand the anatomy. (Fig. 6.21)

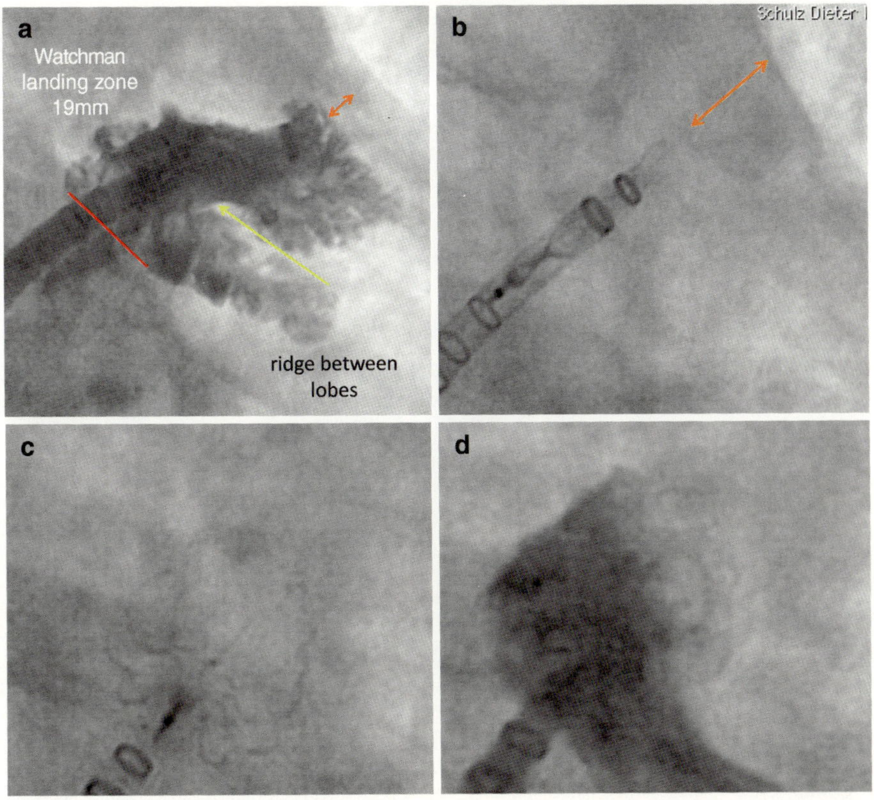

Fig. 6.21 Case 5: successful closure of a dual lobe LAA in RAO caudal projection. (**a**) Watchman guiding is positioned in the upper lobe. (**b**) Watchman release is started just distal to the interridge. (**c**) Position of the Watchman 24 mm device after release. (**d**) Angiographic documentation of closure

- device release is started from the upper lobe, sufficiently proximal so that the Watchman can unfold and cover the inferior lobe. (Fig. 6.21)
- echo assessment of the result including colour flow (Fig. 6.22)

6.1.6 LAA with Single Lobe (Case 6)

Learning objectives: strategy for sizing and occluding single lobe LAA.

The LAA does not seem difficult since the anatomy is quite straight forward (Fig. 6.23). The oversized 24 mm device fits well into the anatomy.

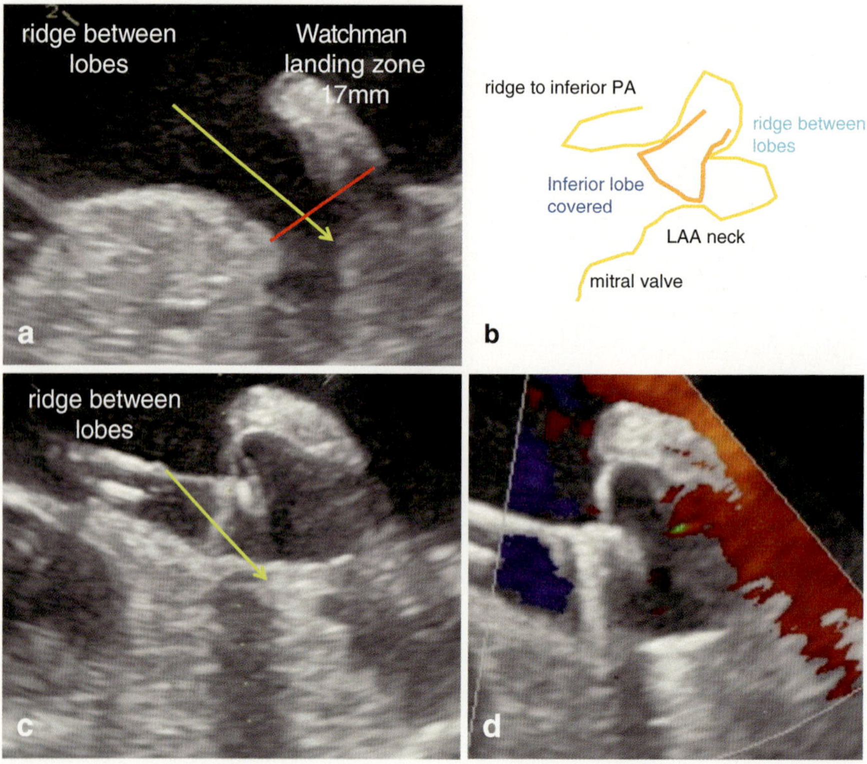

Fig. 6.22 Case 5: successful closure of a dual lobe LAA with a proximal ridge (**a**) Echo visualization of proximal Watchman landing zone. (**b**) Schematic illustration of LAA closure technique employing the Watchman with this particular anatomy. (**c**) Watchman position after release: anchoring of the device in the anterior lobe, proximal part covers the entrance to the inferior lobe. (**d**) Position of the Watchman 24 mm device after release with colour flow. No gap >5 mm is observed

- measurement of landing zone by angiography and echo measurements suggests a 24 mm device (Fig. 6.23)
- following release, a "shoulder" is noted at 145° measuring 10 mm.
- all PASS criteria are fulfilled, the device can be detached from the delivery cable (Fig. 6.24)

6.1.7 *Multilobe LAA (Case 7)*

Learning objective: large, multilobe LAA anatomy requires a proximal position for complete LAA closure.

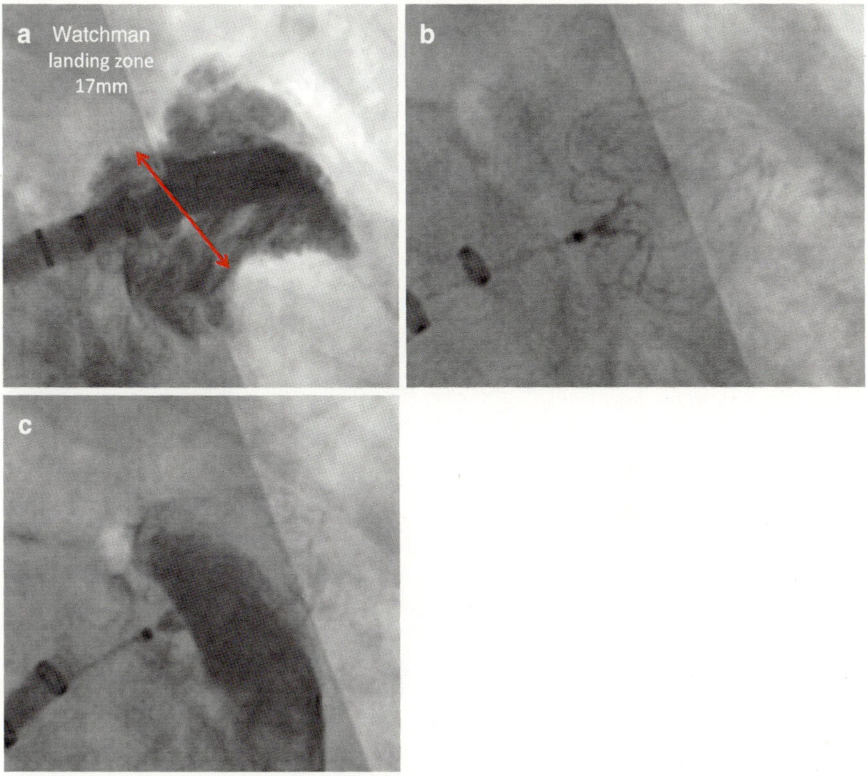

Fig. 6.23 Case 6: successful closure of a single lobe LAA (**a**) RAO caudal visualization of the LAA including the landing zone measurement. (**b**) Watchman 24 mm position after release: anchoring of the device in the depth of the LAA. (**c**) Position of the Watchman 24 mm device after release in angiography

Large anatomies with multiple lobes are defined as broccoli-type anatomy. Once the correct angiographic projection is achieved (mostly RAO 20°, caudal 15° as a starting point), it becomes clear that this LAA has an anterior orientation with multiple shallow lobes. The strategy is to anchor the device in a middle lobe which gives the device a straight orientation towards the proximal landing zone.

- deep positioning of the pigtail allows to completely visualize the LAA (Fig. 6.25)
- 3D reconstruction as well as X-plane visualization of the LAA measures Watchman landing zone to have a maximum diameter of 23 mm leading to a 27 mm device ("2 sizes up", Fig. 6.26)
- First, distal release of the device leaves a gap >5 mm at the inferior end (Fig. 6.27). Note the constrained appearance of the distal part of the Watchman device reflecting the anatomy of that particular lobe employed for anchoring.

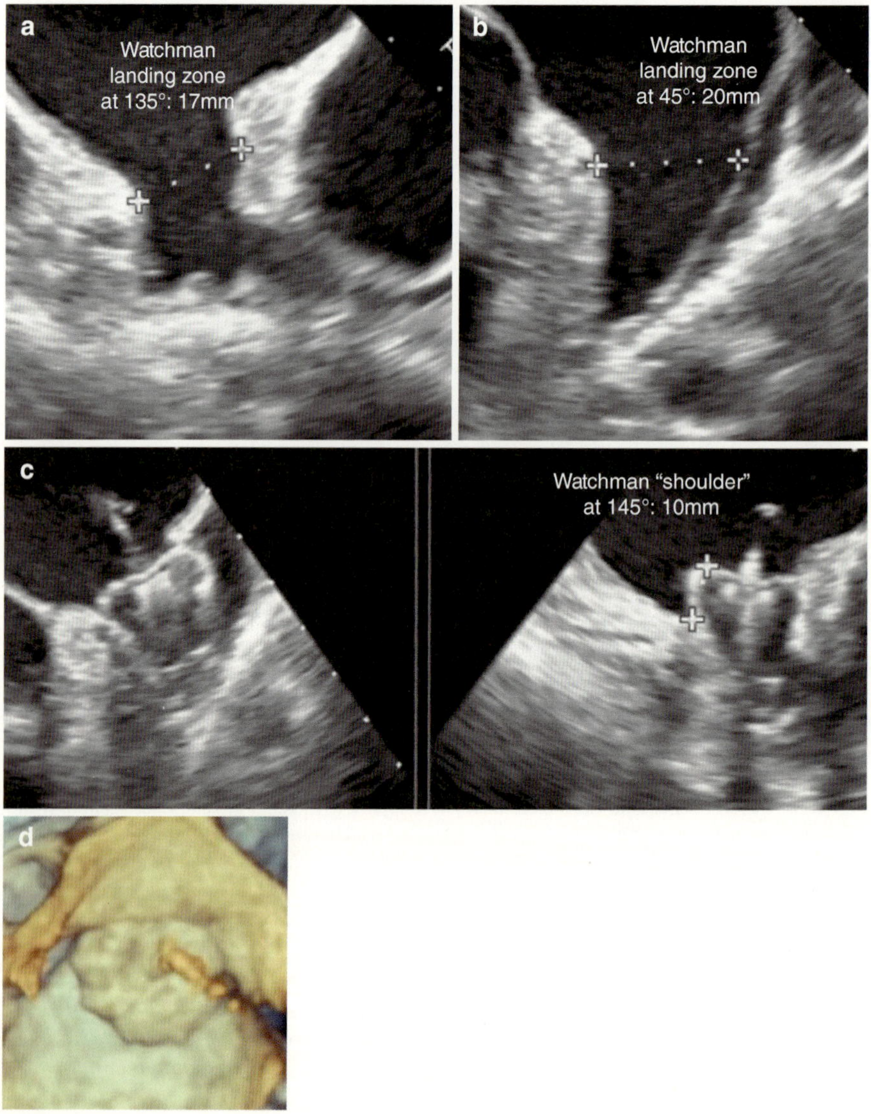

Fig. 6.24 Case 6: successful closure of a single lobe LAA (**a**) echo visualization of LAA including landing zone at 135° corresponding to RAO caudal projection. (**b**) Watchman 24 mm position after release: anchoring of the device in the depth of the LAA (**c**) Watchman 24 mm position after release in X-plane 45/135°: anchoring of the device in the depth of the LAA, inferior shoulder <40% of device height (**d**) 3D imaging of complete LAA closure

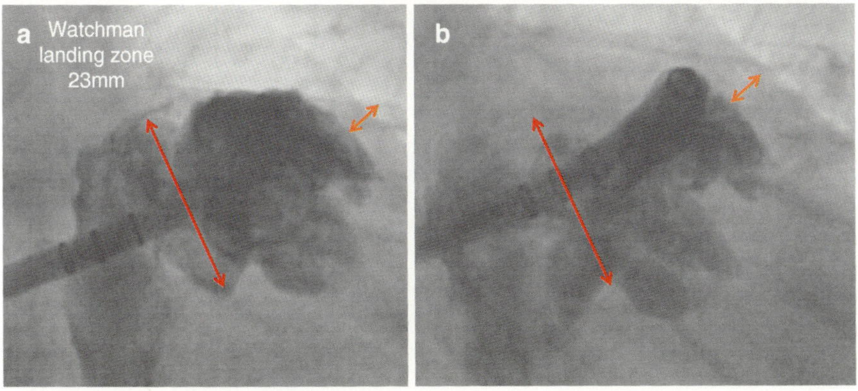

Fig. 6.25 Case 7: successful closure of a multiple lobed LAA (**a**) Angiographic imaging of LAA including landing zone diameter measurement. According to the measurements a 27 mm device was chosen (**b**) Employing the pigtail as a rail, the sheath is positioned deep into the LAA. Now the 27 mm mark on the sheath (middle ring) is located at the landing zone.

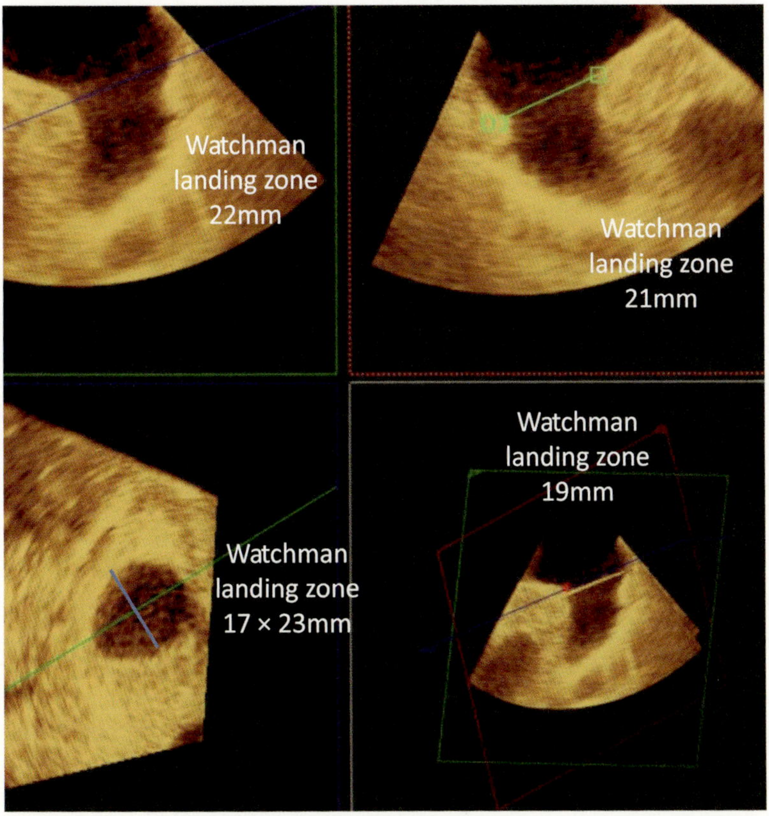

Fig. 6.26 Case 7: 3D reconstruction of the LAA Watchman landing zone employing the Q-lab software. Oval shape ostium of the LAA, largest diameter measured is 23 mm leading to a 27 mm Watchman device size

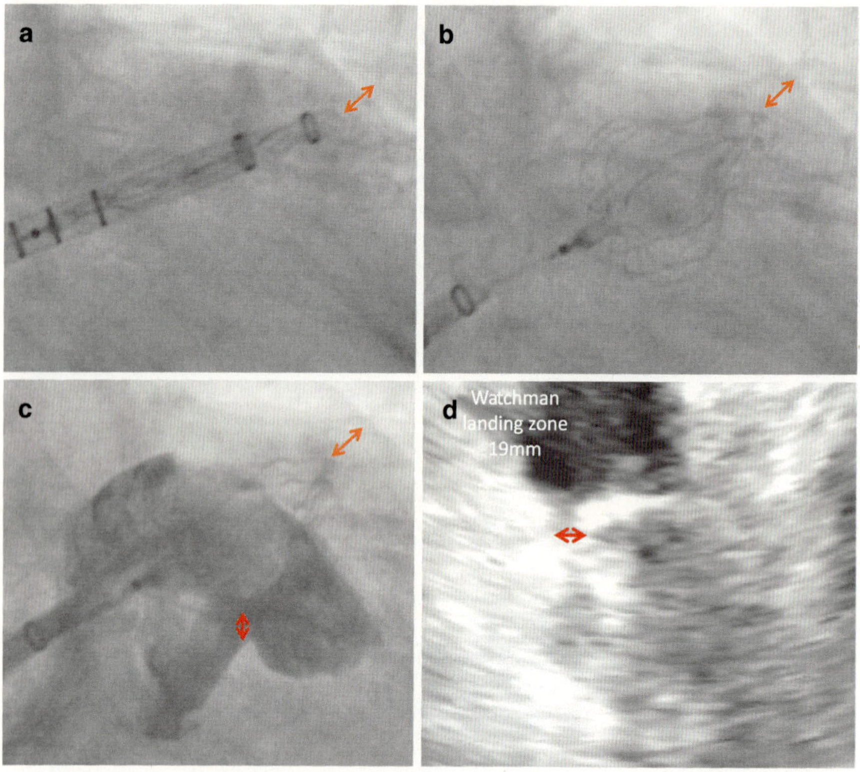

Fig. 6.27 Case 7: distal release leads to a gap. (**a**) The device is released at the distal part of the LAA. Note the orange arrow marking the distance to pericardial shadow. (**b**) After release, the distal part of the device is highly compressed. (**c**) large inferior gap to the lower lobe in angiography and echocardiography (**c**, **d**)

- Partial recapture of the device and second release more proximal; orientation is given by the epicardial boarder. Note the change in shape of the Watchman now appearing more "classical" (Fig. 6.28).
- angiographic and echocardiographic criteria see the device to completely cover the LAA (Fig. 6.28).

6.1.8 *Multilobe, Large LAA and Transseptal Puncture (Broccoli-Type, Case 8)*

Learning objective: Broccoli-type anatomy with large proximal landing zone and multiple, shallow distal lobes requires device anchoring in a middle lobe.

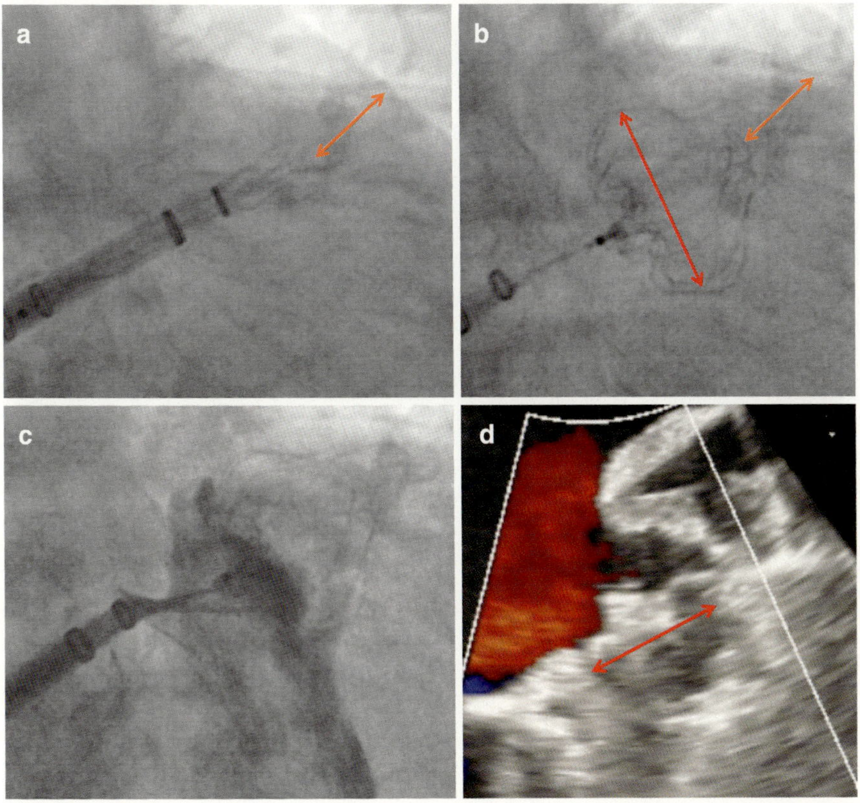

Fig. 6.28 Case 7: partial recapture and proximal release leads to complete closure. (**a**) The device is partially recaptured. (**b**) Employing the shadow of the epicardium for orientation, the device release is started more proximally. After this maneuver, the LAA is closed completely as seen in angiography and echocardiography (**c**, **d**)

The LAA anatomy of this particular case is challenging from first glance at the anatomy: multiple shallow lobes with a large ostium measured at 29 mm both in angiography and echo (Figs. 6.29, 6.30 and 6.31, echo not shown). This case illustrates the flexibility of the Watchman device and the importance of low and inferior transseptal puncture.

- The initial location of the transseptal puncture results in a torqued access to the LAA of the Watchman sheath, which limits control of the 33 mm Watchman device during release (Fig. 6.29a–c). While device release was started in the upper lobe (Fig. 6.29b), the device immediately loses distal anchoring upon release and dislocates into an unacceptable, non-sealing position in the inferior lobe (Fig. 6.29c, d).

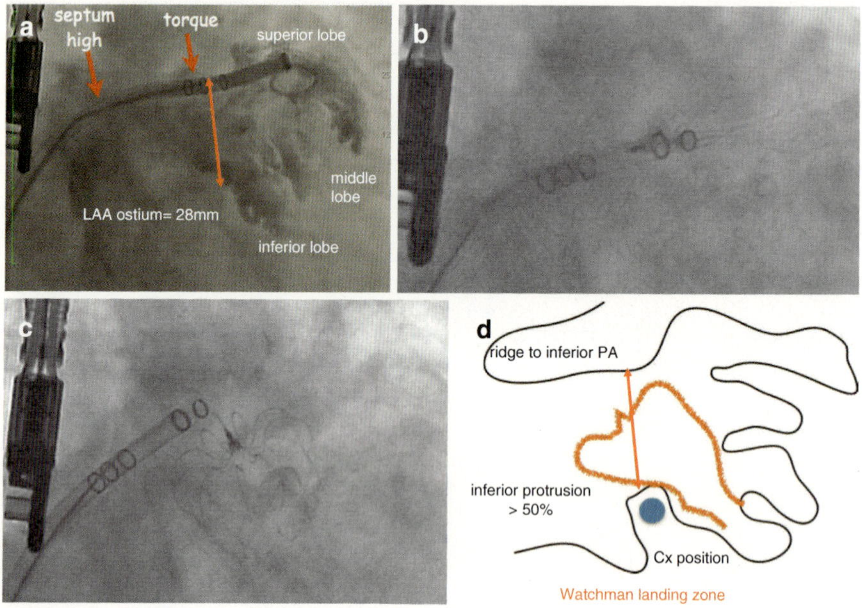

Fig. 6.29 Case 8: RAO caudal view during a complex LAA closure. Large LAA with initially high transseptal puncture and torqued access of the Watchman sheath (**a**). Although release of the Watchman device is started in the anterior, superior LAA lobe (**b**) the device falls into the inferior lobe upon release. The 33 mm Watchman does not cover the LAA ostium and shows a huge, unacceptable protrusion into the left atrium. **c** + **d**

- The decision is made to perform a second more inferior and posterior transseptal puncture (Fig. 6.30a). This leads to a much better control of the orientation of the Watchman sheath which now can be positioned in the distal part of the superior and anterior LAA lobe (Fig. 6.30b).
- The first device release now has the 33 mm device only in the upper lobe (Fig. 6.30c); the anatomy would not allow the large device to open up and cover the inferior lobes in this distal position.
- A second attempt is made with the device in the inferior lobe—a large shoulder and a gap towards the superior lobe is observed (Fig. 6.31d).
- Finally the device release is started with the Watchman sheath located in a "middle" lobe. Already the shape of the device now looks ideal "strawberry-like", also the tug test is ok with no movement of the device (Fig. 6.32). Both the angiography (Fig. 6.32c) and the echo (not shown) finds release criteria compression (size), position and seal to be correct.

Using the middle lobe of a broccoli-type LAA for distal anchoring was found to lead to successful closure in several cases. Alternatively a superior lobe with the device sitting very proximal has proven to be a successful strategy. Anchoring the

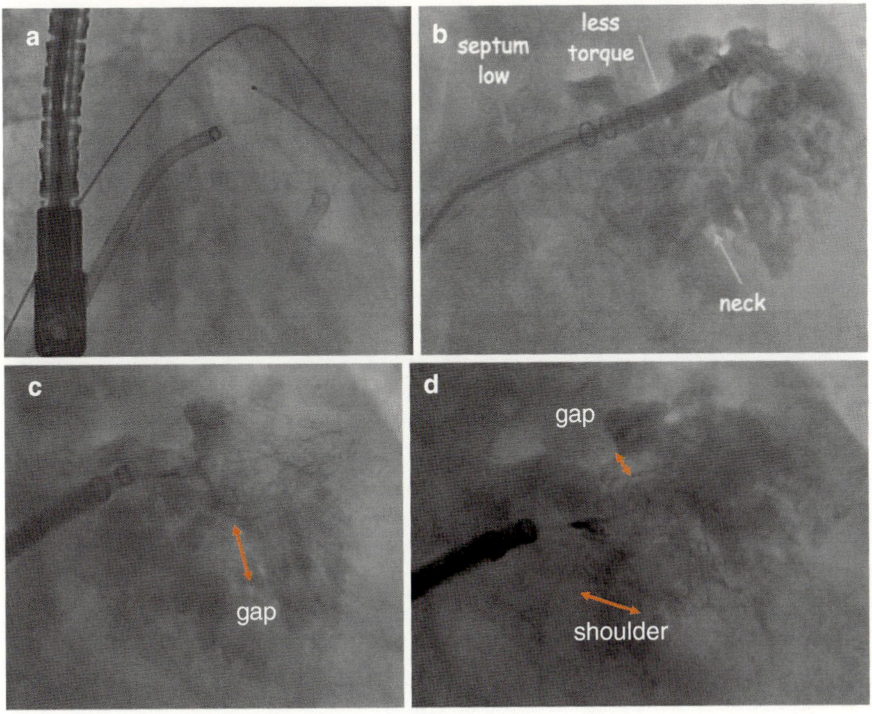

Fig. 6.30 Case 8: RAO caudal view of LAA closure in a broccoli-type LAA anatomy. A second more inferior transseptal puncture is performed (**a**). This allows to access the depth of the LAA with less torque in the Watchman sheath over the pigtail (**b**). First release of the 33 mm Watchman is too distal, the device is entrapped in the upper lobe and does not cover the inferior lobe(**c**). After partial recapture and release of the device in the inferior lobe, a gap >5 mm is observed towards the superior lobe (**d**)

device in an inferior lobe always leads to large shoulders with unacceptable protrusion of the device into the left atrium. In addition, inferior transseptal puncture and device oversizing by 20% or more has proven to be key to successful LAA closure particularly in this anatomy.

6.1.9 *Large LAA Closed by Two Devices ("Kissing Watchman", Case 9)*

Learning objective: LAA ostium may be larger than 30 mm; currently no device is available to cover such a large landing zone.

Currently the largest landing zone covered by the available devices is 30 mm. Some LAA are even larger than these measurements. Several operators have

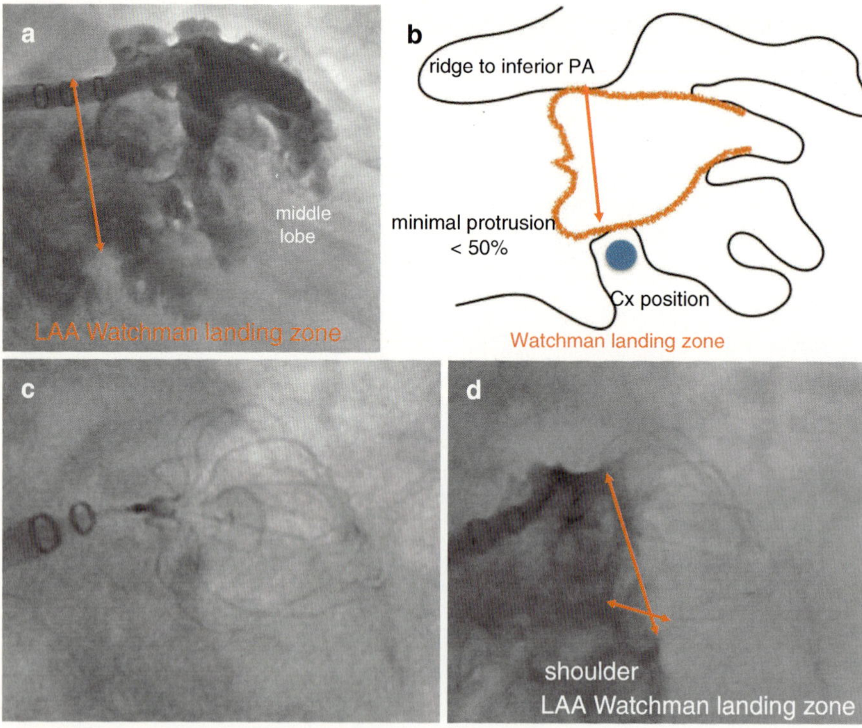

Fig. 6.31 Case 8: RAO caudal view of LAA closure in a broccoli-type LAA anatomy. Final position with the distal part of the 33 mm Watchman device anchored in the middle lobe slightly more proximal than the release position shown in Fig. 5.35c (**a**) initial imaging of the broccoli-type LAA anatomy. Angiographic landing zone is depicted. (**b**) schematic drawing of the strategy for successful closure of this type of anatomy. The device is anchored in a middle lobe and spans the whole ostium. (**c**) Final position of Watchman anchored in a middle lobe. Compared to the initial image of the LAA in the same projection (**a**), the device now spans the entire ostium with no angiographic leakage (**d**). This observation was confirmed by echo (images not shown). This leads to complete sealing of this particularly challenging LAA anatomy

described the option of single lobe closure employing two devices; of note, this is clearly outside of the device instructions for use but it is the only option for these patients as no larger devices are currently available.

- Echocardiographic and angiographic measurements find the landing zone to be between 32 and 34 mm; two large lobes measuring around 18 mm and 19 mm are visualized by angiography (Fig. 6.32)
- A 21 mm device is positioned first in the inferior lobe (Fig. 6.33a)

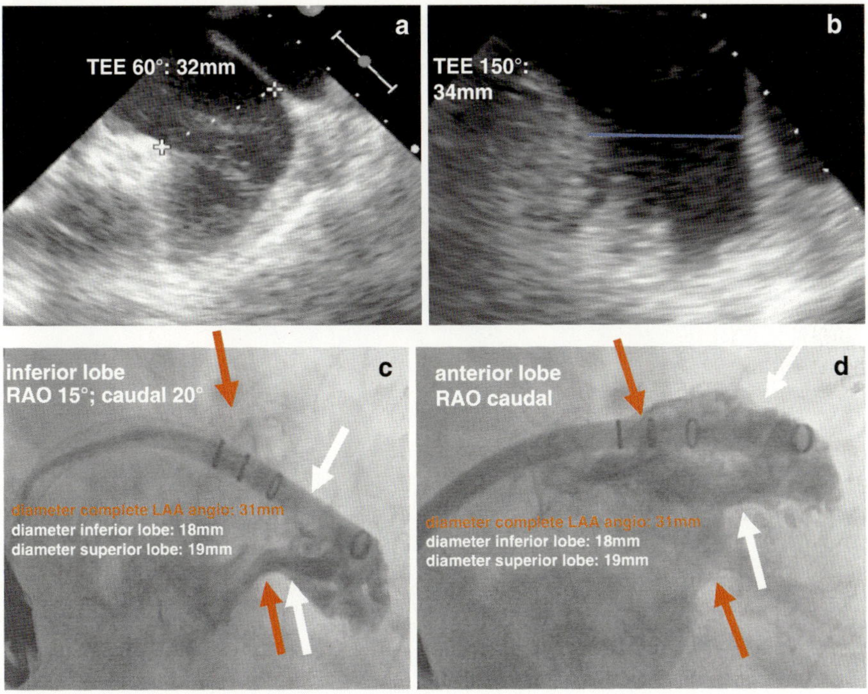

Fig. 6.32 Case 9: "Kissing" Watchman. The echo images show a LAA with a proximal Watchman landing zone of 32–34 mm. This diameter is too large to be covered by a single endoluminal device device (**a**, **b**). Probing and visualizing the depth of the LAA with the pigtail confirms two lobes with a proximal diameter of 18–19 mm each (**c**, **d**)

- a second 21 mm device is positioned in the superior lobe (Fig. 6.33c)
- echocardiographic and angiographic assessment finds the devices to successfully close the two lobes (Figs. 6.33 and 6.34)

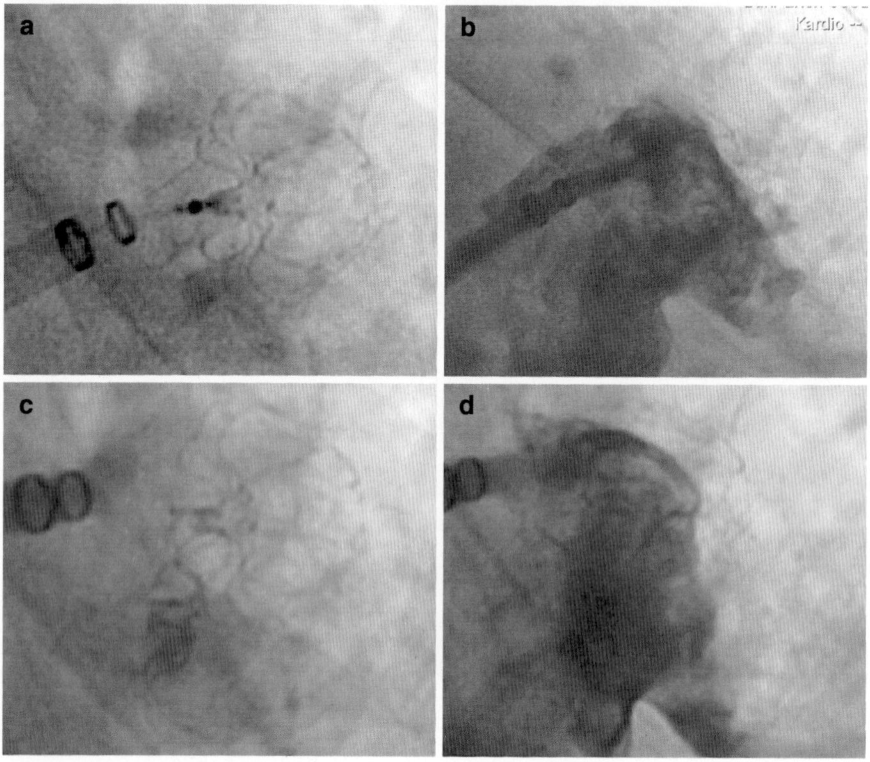

Fig. 6.33 Case 9: the two lobes are closed with a 21 mm Watchman each; first the sheath engages the depth of the anterior lobe (**a**, **b**), then a 21 mm Watchman device is deployed in the inferior lobe. Final angiography confirms complete closure of the LAA (**c**, **d**)

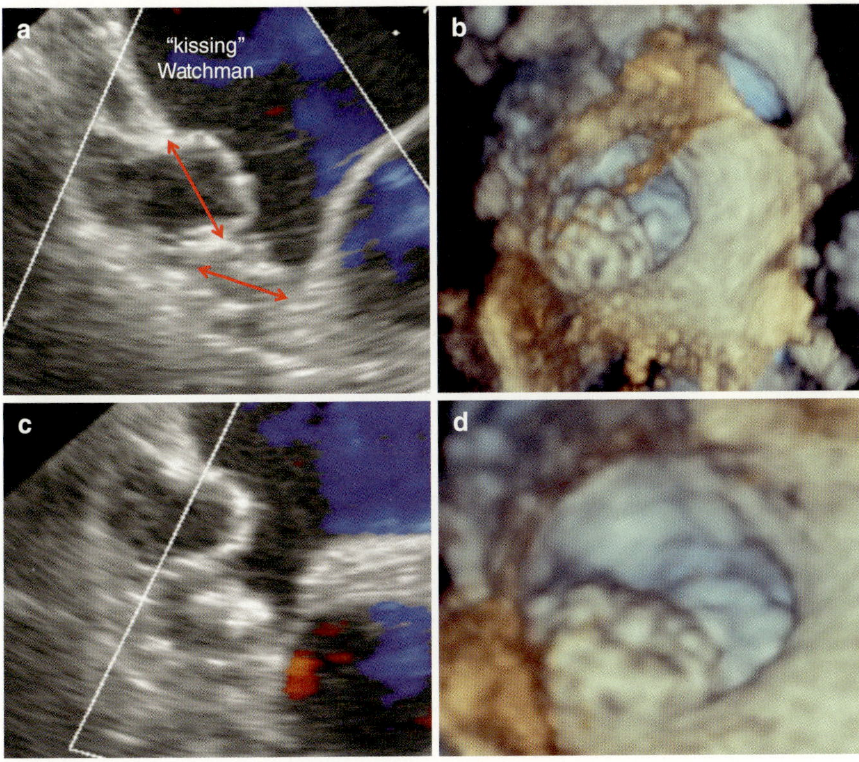

Fig. 6.34 Case 9: echocardiographic imaging confirms that both lobes are completely sealed. (**a**, **c**) No colour flow is seen around the device. The 3D images demonstrate that the occluder in medial position overlaps the device that is positioned in the more laterally located lobe (**b**, **d**)

Acknowledgment The authors would like to thank Mrs. Elisa Vireca, MS, Boston Scientific, Diegem, Belgium for critical reading and helpful comments.

Chapter 7
Amplatzer Amulet Implantation

7.1 Device Features

The Amplatzer Amulet is a nitinol wire mesh self-expanding device with a distal lobe and a proximal disc, which are connected by a flexible waist (Fig. 7.1). The lobe of the device has 6–10 pairs of stabilizing wires and is implanted in the proximal 10–15 mm of the left atrial appendage (LAA), whereas the disc of the device is intended to cover the left atrial side of the LAA. There are eight different device sizes from 16 to 34 mm, based on the width of the device lobe (Fig. 7.2) [1]. The Amplatzer Amulet is suitable for implantation in a LAA landing zone (neck) diameter of between 11 and 31 mm, and a LAA depth of at least 12 mm.

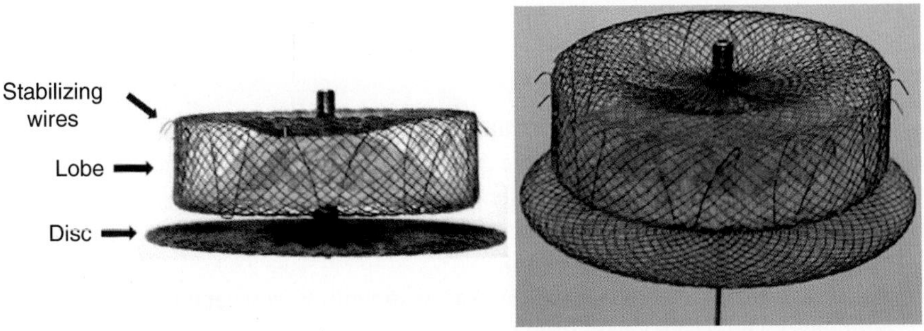

Fig. 7.1 The Amplatzer Amulet device consists of a distal lobe and a proximal disc, which are connected by an articulated waist. The lobe has 6–10 pairs of stabilizing wires to securely anchor the device in the LAA

M.W. Bergmann et al., *Clinical Cases in LAA Occlusion*,
DOI 10.1007/978-3-319-51431-4_7

AMPLATZER AMULET SIZING CHART

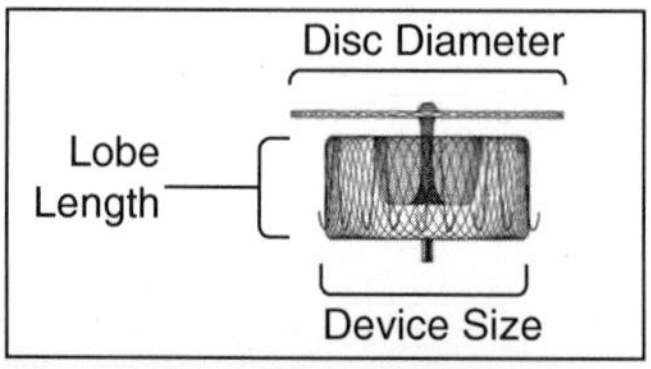

Maximum Landing Zone Width (mm)	Amulet™ Device Size	Lobe Length (mm)	Minimum LAA Depth (mm)	Disc Diameter (mm)	Sheath Diameter
11.0 – 13.0	**16**	7.5	≥10	22	12 F *or* 14 F (with adaptor)
13.0 – 15.0	**18**	7.5	≥10	24	
15.0 – 17.0	**20**	7.5	≥10	26	
17.0 – 19.0	**22**	7.5	≥10	28	
19.0 – 22.0	**25**	10	≥12	32	
22.0 – 25.0	**28**	10	≥12	35	14 F
25.0 – 28.0	**31**	10	≥12	38	
28.0 – 31.0	**34**	10	≥12	41	

Fig. 7.2 There are eight different sizes of Amplatzer Amulet devices, which can be divided to two groups: devices 16–22 mm that have a shorter (7.5 mm) lobe length and devices 25–34 mm that have a longer (10mm) lobe length. The smaller devices usually require more oversizing. When using large Amulet devices, especially in LAAs with a small ostium and a large neck, the distance from the mitral valve should be evaluated before and after device implantation to avoid any potential impingement

7.2 Step by Step

7.2.1 Before Puncture

- Usually, the patient is under general anesthesia or conscious sedation due to the discomfort from the use of intraprocedural TEE. Intracardiac echocardiography (ICE) may be also used with excellent success.
- At the beginning, TEE is performed to exclude thrombus, which is usually a contraindication to perform LAAO.
- The baseline status of the pericardial space, the mitral valve and the left superior pulmonary vein (LSPV) are briefly assessed.
- The LAA is scanned from 0° to 135° and the maximum and minimum diameters of the ostium and the landing zone are recorded (Fig. 7.3a–c). Real time 3D TEE may allow for better spatial visualization of the LAA and more comprehensive evaluation of the device during the procedure (Fig. 7.3d).
- The use of multislice computed tomography (MSCT) prior to the procedure will also facilitate procedural planning as it has higher spatial resolution and is less operator-dependent than TEE.

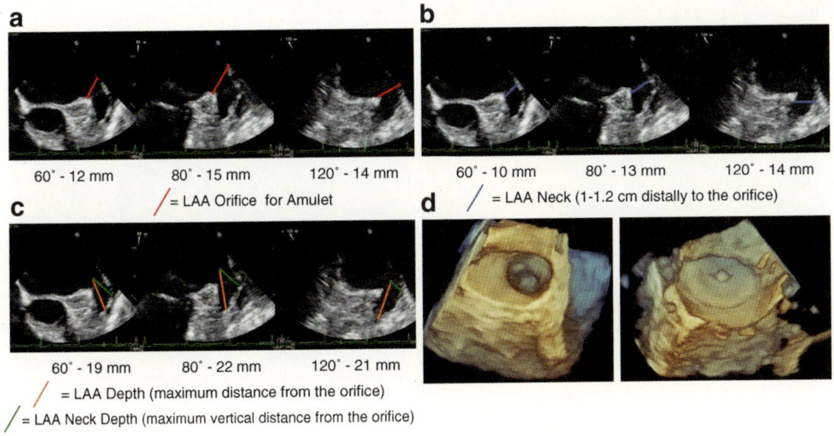

Fig. 7.3 Echocardiographic scanning from 0 to 135 degrees is recommended before Amplatzer Amulet implantation to evaluate the dimensions of the LAA ostium and neck. The LAA neck definition (*blue line*) is different than the one used for the Watchman device and is measured 12 mm distal to the LAA ostium (*red line*). Also the LAA depth definition is different: for Amulet a line perpendicular to the LAA ostium (*green line*) is used, whereas for Watchman a line from the ostium to the tip of a distal lobe is used (*orange line*)

7.2.2 *Vascular Access: Transseptal Puncture*

- The right femoral vein is punctured using standard technique.
- Transseptal puncture (TSP) is performed under fluoroscopic and TEE guidance in the infero-posterior portion of the fossa ovalis.
- Unfractionated heparin is given in a dose of 100 IU/kg to obtain an activated clotting time (ACT) of 250–300 s. Giving a half dose of heparin before TSP provides some antithrombotic protection in case of a difficult or prolonged TSP.

7.2.3 *Device Sizing*

- A selective injection of contrast in a right anterior oblique (RAO) 30°/cranial 20° view and in a RAO 30°/caudal 20° view is performed through the transseptal sheath with a 5–6 French (F) marker pigtail catheter sitting inside the LAA (Fig. 7.4).
- Device sizing is based on multimodality imaging (TEE, angiography and/or MSCT).

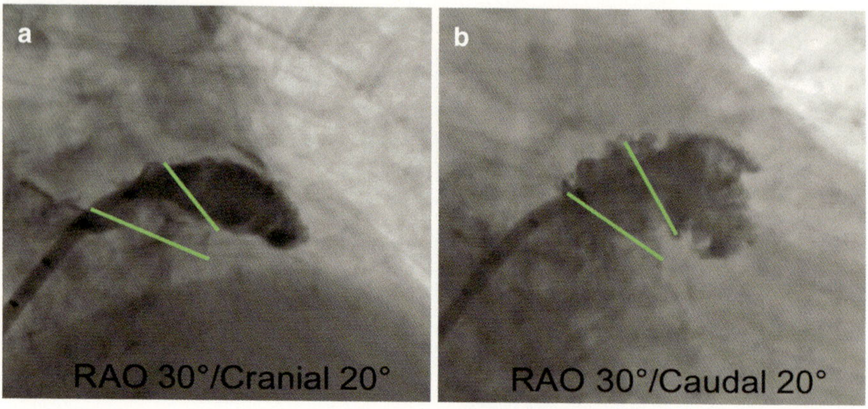

Fig. 7.4 The LAA ostium is more clearly visible on RAO Cranial views (Fig 7.4a) whereas the distal part of LAA is better depicted in RAO Caudal views (Fig. 7.4b)

- Amulet needs to be oversized in relation to the maximum dimensions of the landing zone (Fig. 7.2) but the device should be less oversized in oval LAA anatomies.
- Amulet sizes 16–22 mm have a shorter lobe (7.5 mm) and waist length (5.5 mm) than sizes 25–34 mm (lobe length of 10 mm, waist length of 8 mm). Therefore, slightly more oversizing (1–2 mm more than the sizing chart recommendation) is preferred when using a smaller Amulet.
- The delivery sheath size, either 12 or 14F, depends on the device size and is chosen based on the sizing chart, (Fig. 7.2). Some operators use the 14F delivery sheath for all cases

7.2.4 Device Preparation

- Device preparation is performed according to the instructions for use. A step-by-step device preparation video is available online (www.laamentor.com).

7.2.5 Stiff Wire: Sheath Exchange

- The safest way to exchange the TSP sheath for the delivery sheath is in the LSPV (or with an Inoue type wire loop in the LA).

- Most operators prefer a 260 cm Amplatz Super Stiff J wire with a short (3 cm) soft tip or a Backup wire (both Boston Scientific, Minneapolis, MN, USA). An alternative is the 260 cm Supercore wire (Abbott).

7.2.6 Device Introduction and Deployment

- The device is introduced into the delivery sheath in a wet-to-wet manner to avoid air embolization and is advanced up to the tip of the sheath.
- Slight retraction of the sheath while holding the delivery cable stable partially exposes the device in the so-called "ball" position (Fig. 7.5). Further slight pushing of the delivery cable produces the "triangular" shape and then the fully deployed lobe.
- Engagement of the delivery sheath within the LAA using a pigtail catheter as in a Watchman implantation has been the standard approach but more recently it has been replaced by the extrusion of the lobe as a ball in the left atrium and then careful intubation in the LAA under TEE guidance (Fig. 7.6, panel a)
- Usually, a counterclockwise rotation of the sheath is needed to orientate the delivery sheath co-axial to the LAA neck (Fig. 7.6, panel b).
- When reaching the optimal position in the landing zone, the sheath is stabilized and the delivery cable advanced and the device lobe deployment is completed (Fig. 7.6, panel c).
- Tensing (pulling slightly) the delivery cable while unsheathing deploys the device disc, allowing it to apply gentle tension to the device lobe and cover the LAA ostium at the left atrial side (Fig. 7.6, panel d).

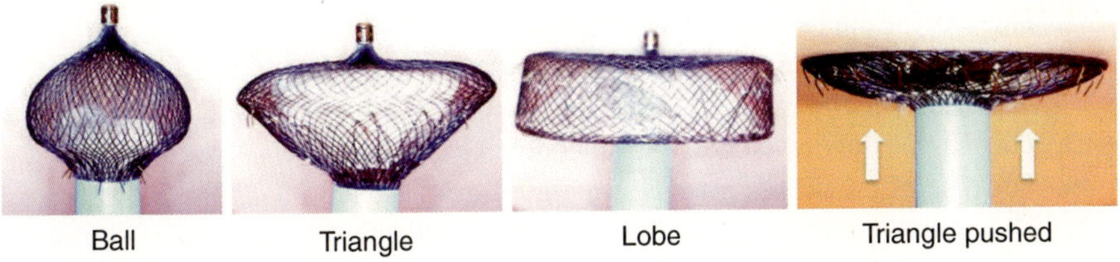

Fig. 7.5 The ball position is achieved by unsheathing the device, i.e. holding the delivery wire stable with one hand and simultaneously pulling the delivery sheath backwards. The device should not be pulled back in the sheath after this stage because the stabilizing wires may damage the tip of the sheath. The device is implanted by pushing the delivery wire from thc ball to the lobe position. An intermediate position is the triangle shape that has the advantage of being almost 100% atraumatic when pushed against the LAA walls. The triangle shape can facilitate deep engagement of the device lobe in the LAA. Also, in the "pushed triangle" shape, the stabilizing wires that are located in the distal part of the device lobe are exposed and can be used for anchoring in difficult LAA anatomies (i.e. inverted chicken wing)

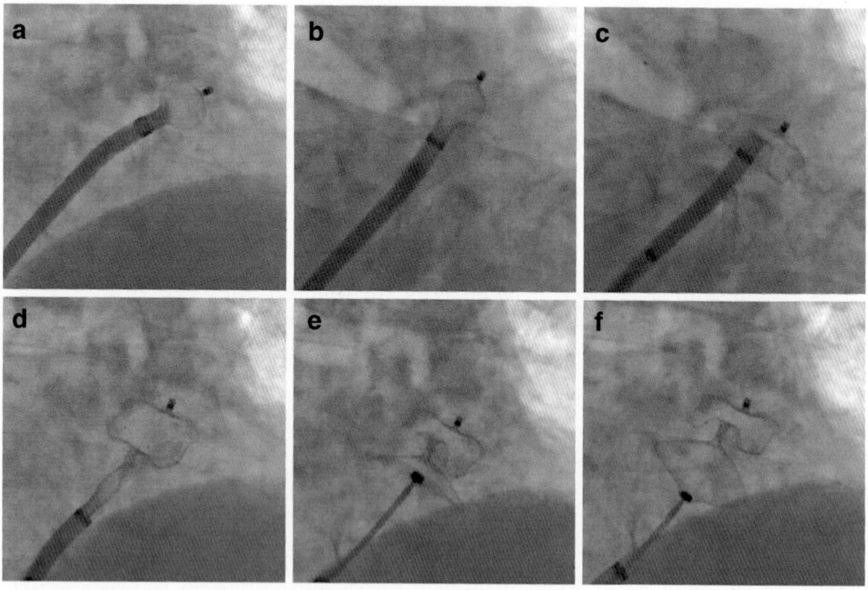

Fig. 7.6 (**a**) Ball position, (**b**) counterclockwise rotation, (**c**) Lobe deployment, (**d**) Disc deployment, (**e**) checking the 5 signs of stability, (**f**) tug test

7.2.7 *Signs of Device Stability, Evaluation of Complete LAAO, Tug Test, and Device Release*

- Five signs of device stability need to be verified prior to release (Fig. 7.6, panel e).
    1. The lobe of the device must be slightly compressed.
    2. The lobe of the device should be oriented perpendicularly to the LAA walls at the level of the neck.
    3. The disc of the device must have a concave shape.
    4. The disc of the device must be separated from the lobe.
    5. The midpoint of the lobe should be distal to the left circumflex coronary artery on TEE.
- The device is checked with color flow TEE from multiple views to confirm the absence of peri-device leaks and optimal coverage of the LAA ostium. Contrast injection can also demonstrate successful LAAO.
- A gentle but sustained (1 minute) tug test to verify device stability is usually performed (Fig. 7.6, panel f).
- The five signs of stability are re-checked and then the device is released by unscrewing the delivery wire (approximately seven counterclockwise rotations).

7.2.8 *Device Recapture: Change*

- Device recapture is done by reversing the steps of deployment. However, the device should not be retracted completely into the sheath as the sheath tip may be damaged or invaginated by the stabilizing wires of the lobe. There is no specific limit in the number of recaptures and deployments but it is very important not to rotate the delivery wire counterclockwise during these maneuvers as this might lead to device embolization.

Acknowledgment The author would like to thank Kevin P. Walsh, Mater Misericordiae University Hospital, Dublin, Ireland for critical reading and helpful comments.

Reference

1. Tzikas A, Gafoor S, Meerkin D, et al. Left atrial appendage occlusion with the AMPLATZER Amulet device: an expert consensus step-by-step approach. EuroIntervention. 2016;11: 1512–21.

Chapter 8
Amplatzer Amulet Implantation: Case Series

8.1 Closure of a Large LAA with a 34 mm Amulet device

Learning objectives: angiographic visualization of the LAA, measurement of landing zone for the distal lobe and proximal disc.

The Amulet can be used to close a LAA that measures 36 mm between the ridge of the pulmonary vein and inferior ostium as shown in this case (Fig. 8.1). The distal lobe needs to be implanted quite deep into the LAA so that the device is stable; too proximal a position results in the device dislocating during the tug test (Fig. 8.2). A

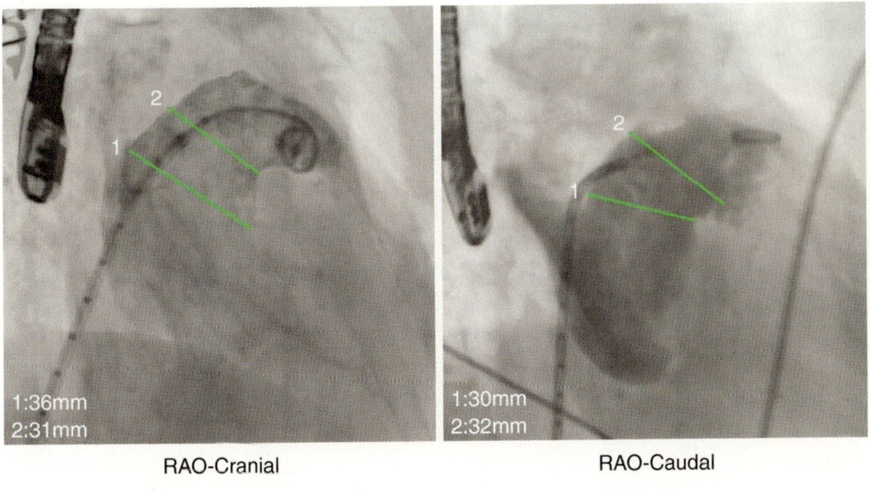

Fig. 8.1 Large LAA closed with Amulet 34 mm: the RAO-Cranial angiography revealed a large LAA with an ostium of 36 mm (*green line* 1) and a landing zone (*neck*) of 31 mm (*green line* 2). The RAO-Caudal view showed an ostium of 30 mm and a landing zone of 32 mm

M.W. Bergmann et al., *Clinical Cases in LAA Occlusion*,
DOI 10.1007/978-3-319-51431-4_8

more distal implantation with the distal lobe taking a triangular shape results in safe anchoring (Fig. 8.3) and good sealing with the proximal disc taking a concave shape (Fig. 8.4).

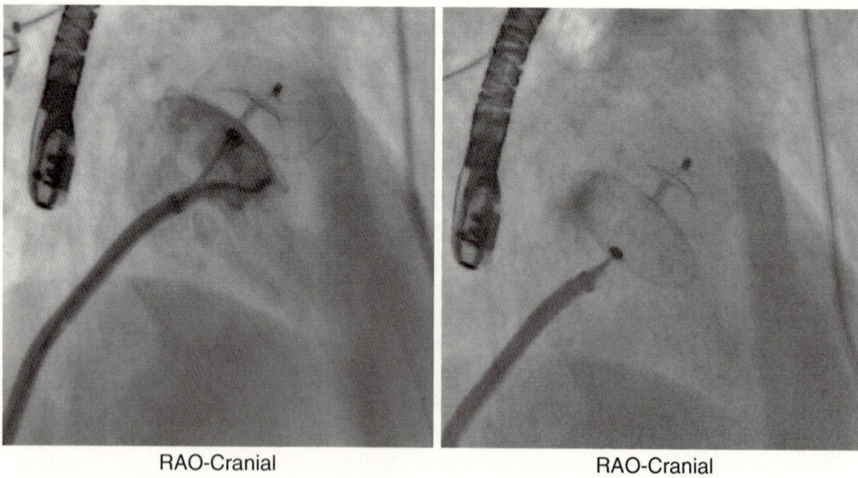

Fig. 8.2 A 34 mm Amulet was implanted. The tug test resulted in device pop-out

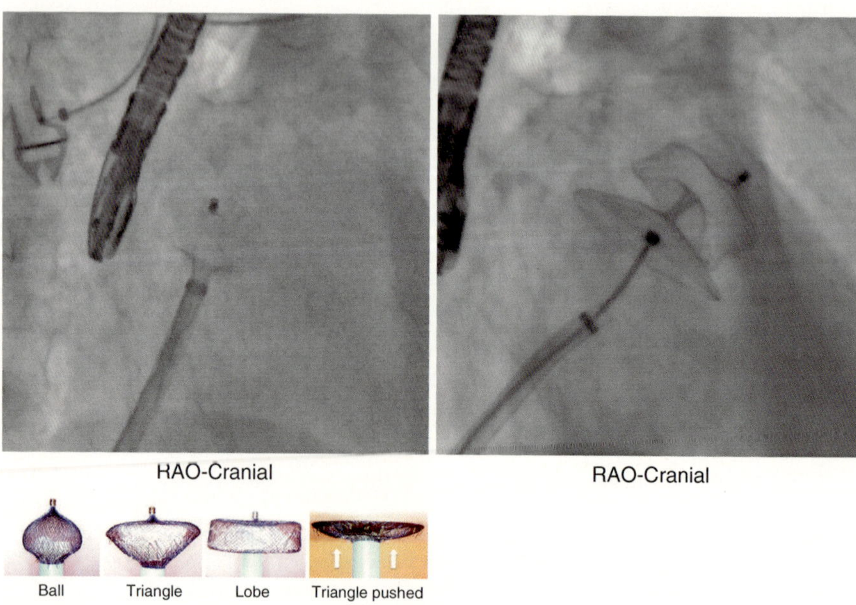

Fig. 8.3 The device was re-positioned deeper using the "triangular shape technique". All five signs of stability were fulfilled

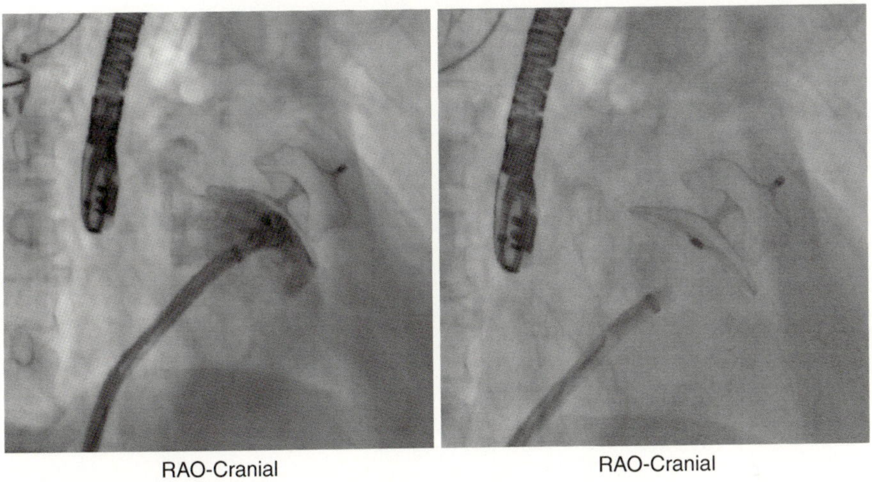

Fig. 8.4 The final angiography showed complete sealing of the LAA

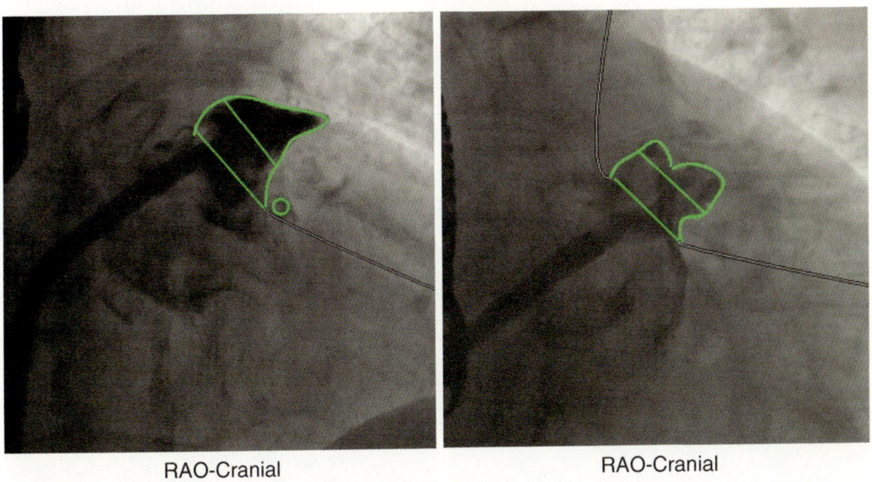

Fig. 8.5 Device embolization of a 25 mm Amulet occluder: angiography in the RAO-Cranial 20 view revealed a relatively shallow funnel shaped LAA. The LCx coronary artery is stented so it can be used as an anatomic landmark on fluoroscopy. Angiography in the RAO-Caudal 20 view reveals a double-lobe shallow LAA. The quality of angiography is suboptimal due to the lack of selective injection

8.2 Closure of a Shallow, Double Lobe LAA with Embolization

Learning objectives: interpret warning signs of device embolization.

The angiography shows a funnel-shaped LAA with two lobes visualized in the RAO caudal projection (Fig. 8.5). As the distal lobe does not anchor adequately (Figs. 8.6 and 8.7) the device embolizes after release (Fig. 8.8).

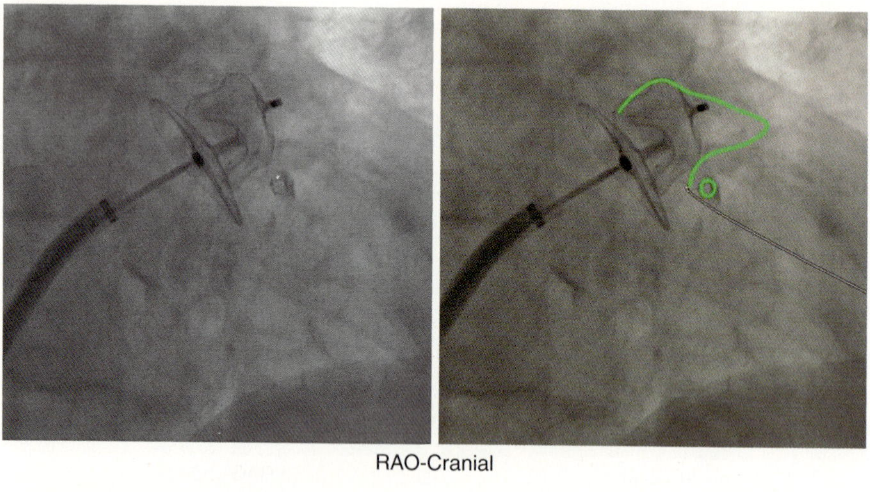

Fig. 8.6 Device embolization: a 25 mm Amulet device was implanted but the device was not placed distally enough. According to the instructions for use (IFU), 2/3 of the device lobe must be placed distal to the LCx artery (this is usually an echocardiographic criterion). In this case the stented LCx artery can be seen on fluoroscopy and the lobe of the device is not deep enough. Moreover, there is no separation between the disc and the lobe and the disc has only a slight concave shape. Device lobe compression and orientation are adequate. Therefore, in this view only 2 out of the 5 signs of stability are visible

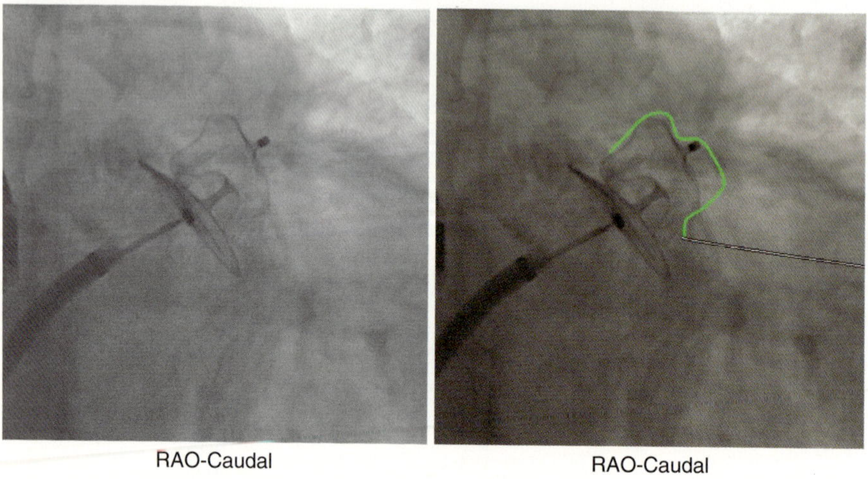

Fig. 8.7 The RAO-Caudal view reveals a shallow implant without lobe-disc separation or a concave shape of the disc. A tug test was performed (not shown) that showed good stability of the device (probably due to the anchoring by the device stabilizing wires) so the device was released

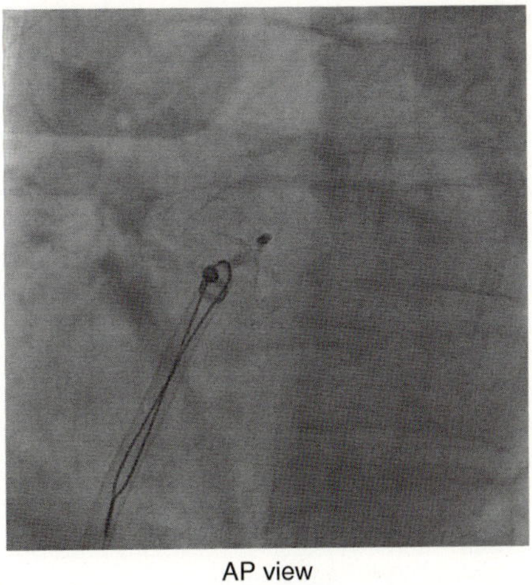

Fig. 8.8 The device embolized immediately after release. It was successfully snared percutaneously without complications

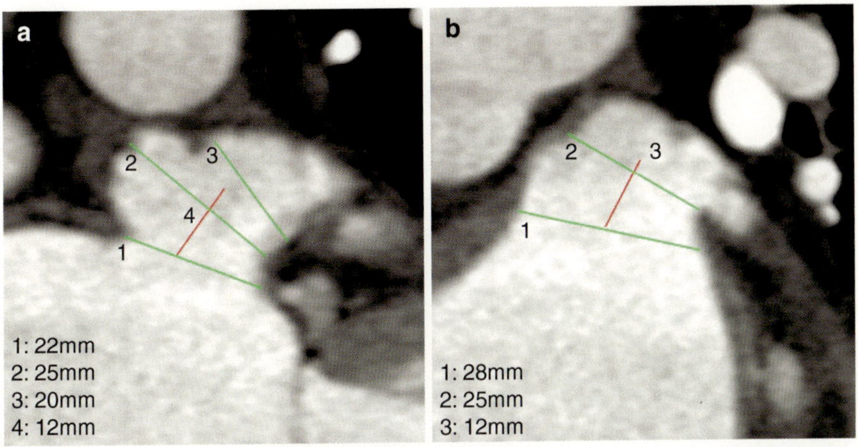

Fig. 8.9 Closure of LAA with an additional small lobe close to its ostium (Amulet 28 mm): pre-procedural MSCT allows for a detailed evaluation of the LAA. Multiplanar reconstruction shows a LAA with a relatively small ostium and an early lobe close to the ostium (panel **a**). The landing zone for the Amulet lobe is 12 mm distal to the ostium (*red line* 4, panel **a**), which is at a "step-down" between *green line* 3 (20 mm) and *green line* 2 (25 mm). In panel **b**, in a different plane, the ostium is larger and the landing zone is 25 mm. In this plane the LAA looks quite shallow. Based on the MSCT data, the patient was judged suitable for an Amulet size of 28 or 31 mm (25 mm landing zone). However, due to the relatively low depth a 28 mm device seemed more appropriate

8.3 LAA with Two Proximal Lobes

Learning objectives: exact positioning of the Amulet device allows for complete sealing.

CT and angiography allow for exact understanding of the anatomy of this particular LAA (Figs. 8.9 and 8.10). Sizing of the distal and proximal landing zones lead to the decision of using a 28 mm Amulet device (Fig. 8.10). An initial release

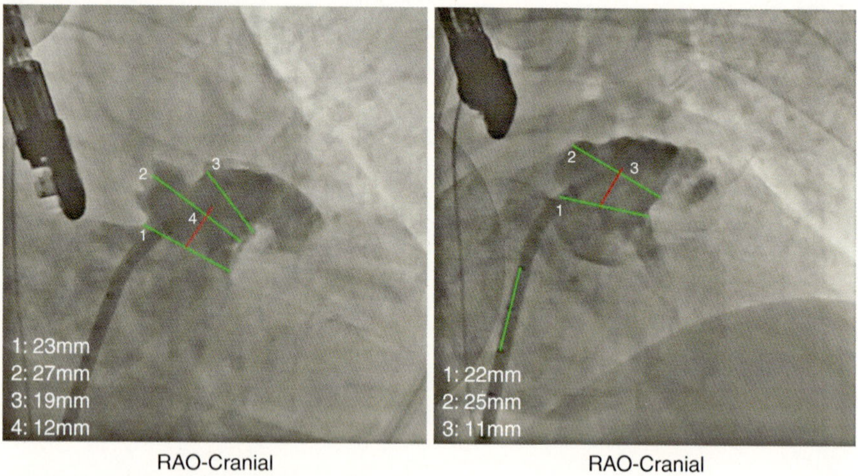

Fig. 8.10 The RAO-Cranial angiography reveals a LAA with an ostium of 23 mm and a landing zone between 19 and 27 mm due to the "step-down" created by the additional early LAA lobe. The RAO-Caudal view shows an ostium of 22 mm and a landing zone of 25 mm. A 28 mm Amulet device is chosen

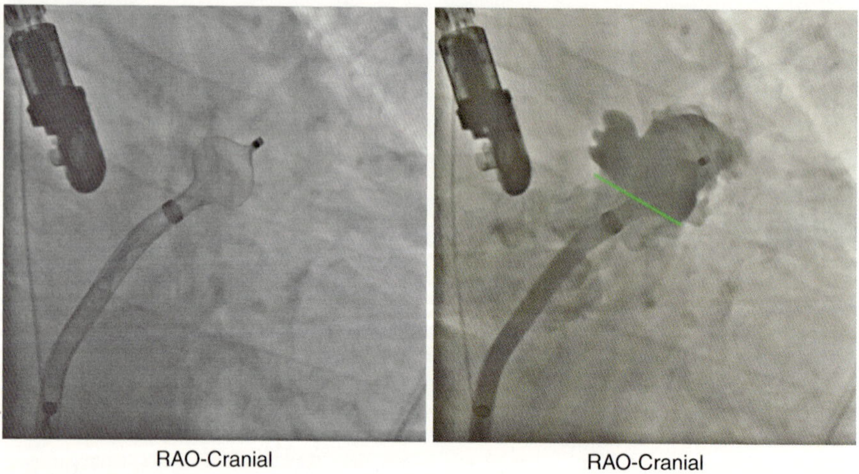

Fig. 8.11 The device is advanced using the ball technique in an RAO-Cranial view. The LAA ostium is denoted by the *green line*

was too proximal (Figs. 8.11 and 8.12), therefore a more distal release was performed (Fig. 8.13). This finally resulted in a good device position with complete closure as judged by angiography (Fig. 8.14) and TEE (not shown). A final prolonged tug test confirmed good device position (Fig. 8.15).

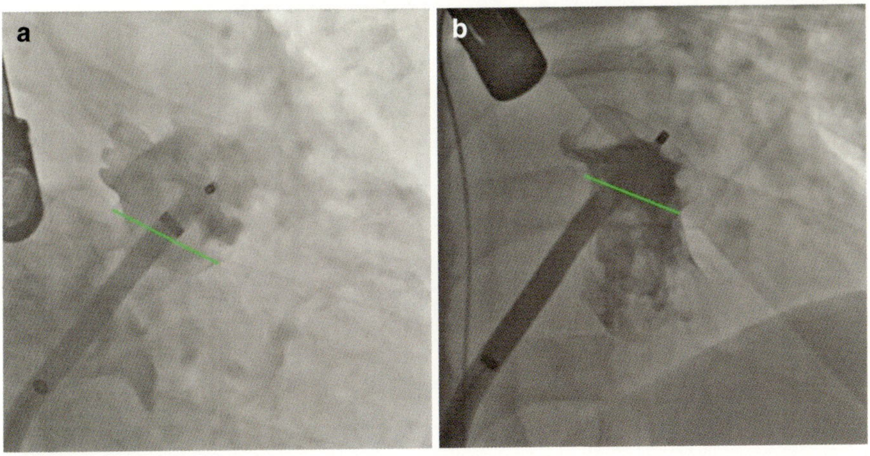

Fig. 8.12 The Amulet lobe deployment is performed. In the Cranial view the device lobe looks off-axis and as if it is protruding into the left atrium. Before deciding to recapture a caudal view was taken, which reveals good device orientation but relatively proximal position of the lobe. The LAA ostium is denoted by the *green line*

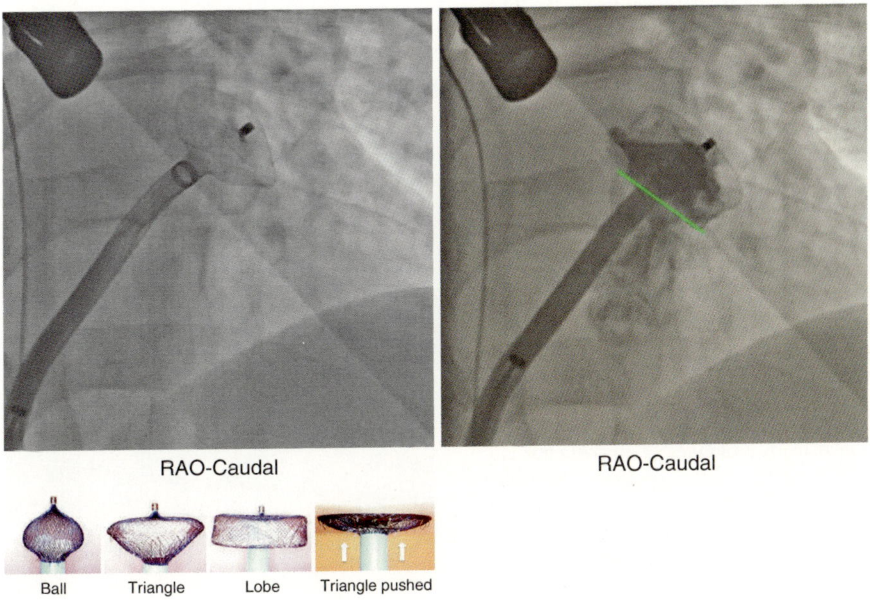

Fig. 8.13 Decision is made to recapture the device and reposition it deeper. The "triangular shape technique" is used in order to advance the device safely deep in the LAA. The final Amulet lobe position is 2 mm deeper than the first one. The LAA ostium is denoted by the *green line*

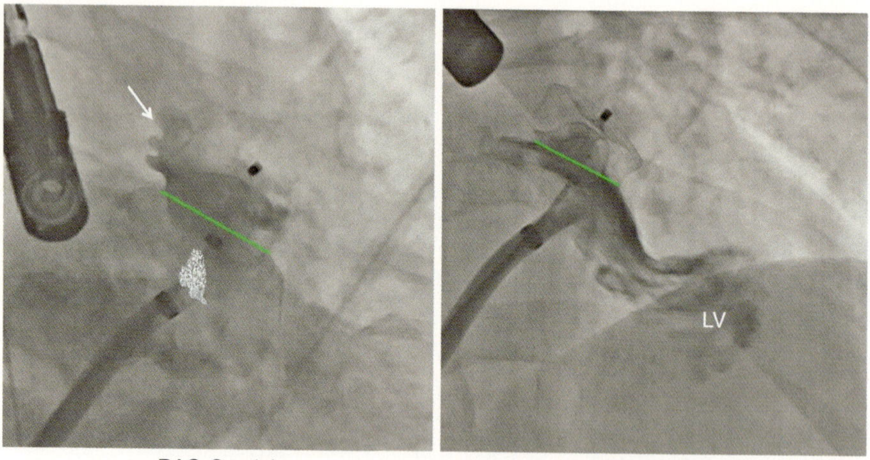

RAO-Cranial RAO-Caudal

Fig. 8.14 Angiography in the RAO-Cranial view showed complete closure of the LAA, except for a small leak that allows contrast to enter the early lobe (*arrow*). The Amulet disc apposition was considered optimal (concave shape, separation between disc and lobe). Good device position is confirmed in the RAO-Caudal view and all 5 signs of device stability are present. In addition, no interference between the device disc and the mitral valve is seen. TEE confirms the findings of angiography. LV—left ventricle

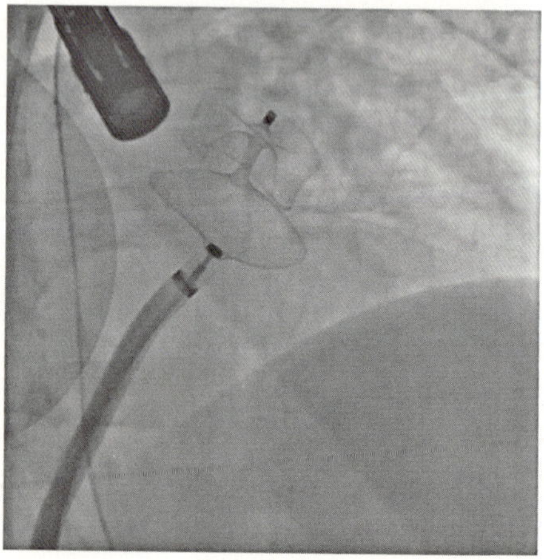

RAO-Caudal

Fig. 8.15 A prolonged (3 min) tug test is performed before final release of the device. Final TEE interrogation reveals no leak in the LAA. No peri-procedural complications occured. TEE at 1 week showed good device position, absence of thrombus, and complete LAA closure

8.4 LAA with Chicken Wing Morphology

Learning objectives: how to negotiate a chicken wing with the Amulet device.

Closure of a LAA with chicken wing morphology requires a special technique. Measurements of the distal and proximal landing zone can be done via MSCT (Fig. 8.16). The 28 mm Amulet is deployed using the ball technique which allows us to push the device distally (Figs. 8.17 and 8.18). Following recapture and a more distal deployment, the device settles in a stable position and the proximal part of the LAA is completely covered (Figs. 8.19 and 8.20).

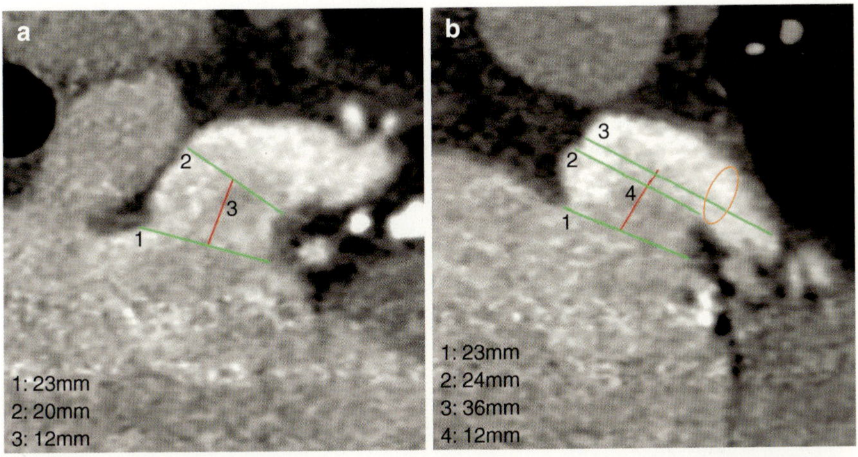

Fig. 8.16 Chicken Wing morphology, Amulet 28 mm with less than optimal transseptal puncture: pre-procedural MSCT allows for a detailed evaluation of the LAA. Multiplanar reconstruction in panel **a** shows a regular LAA with an ostium of 23 mm and a landing zone of 20 mm. In a different view (panel **b**) the LAA has a chicken wing configuration with a short neck (<10 mm). At the level of the landing zone (*red line*, 12 mm distal to the ostium) the width of the LAA is 36 mm (line 3), due to the presence of the "wing". According to panel **a** analysis the patient is suitable for a 25 mm Amulet. However, panel **b** raises questions on whether this LAA should be treated with the "Sandwich Technique", which means to oversize the device and try to implant the Amulet lobe parallel and not vertical to line 3. The key dimension for this decision is the orifice of the "wing" (*orange ellipse*). If this is <10 mm the Amulet lobe cannot fit through so the "Sandwich Technique" is abandoned and the LAA is treated as if there is no "wing". Therefore, with a landing zone of 24 mm, the patient is suitable for a 28 mm Amulet device. The MSCT analysis can help in the decision making but may be influenced by the patient's blood volume/hydration staus. The final decision should be taken by angiography and/or TEE

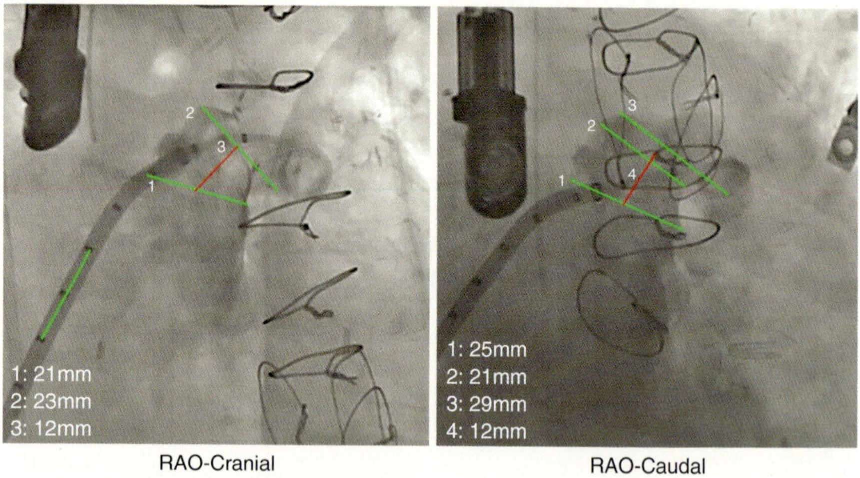

Fig. 8.17 In this patient, venous access from the right groin is blocked so a left femoral vein approach is taken. Due to previous thoracotomy, the heart has an unusual orientation and the interatrial septum is quite rigid. For all these reasons, the transseptal puncture (TSP) is very challenging and the orientation of the catheters and sheath in relation to the LAA is suboptimal. The RAO-Cranial angiography reveals a LAA with an ostium of 21 mm and a landing zone of 23 mm. In the RAO-Caudal view, the "chicken wing" configuration is shown, with a "wing" length of 29 mm. Based on the MSCT analysis and after careful evaluation of the angiography a 28 mm Amulet device is chosen. The aim is to push the Amulet lobe distally in the "wing". From the MSCT analysis it was anticipated that the device lobe would not fit in the "wing"

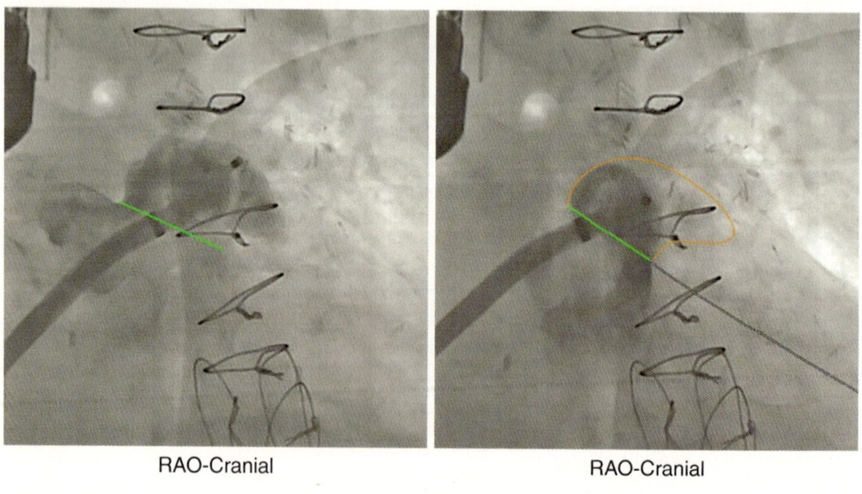

Fig. 8.18 The Amulet lobe is deployed using the ball technique for engaging in the LAA. In the RAO-Cranial view, the orientation of the lobe is not optimal. The main reason for this is the suboptimal TSP. The LAA ostium is denoted by the *green line* and the LAA body by the *orange line*

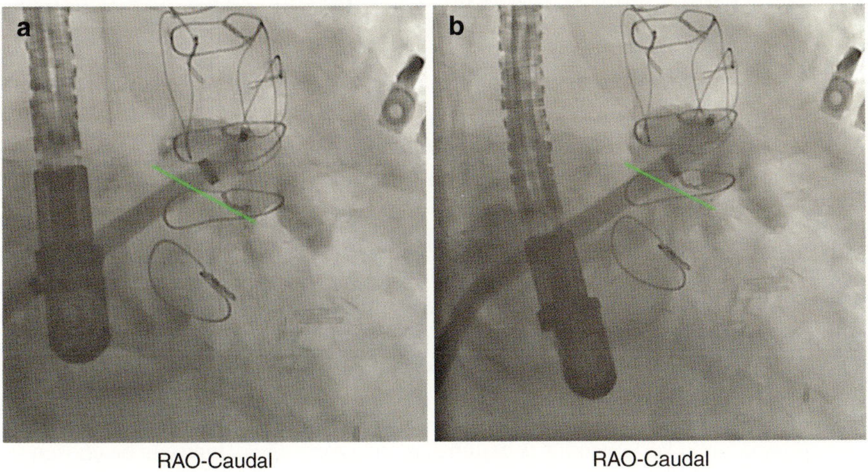

Fig. 8.19 The suboptimal TSP is nicely depicted in the RAO-Caudal view. Although a full counterclockwise rotation of the delivery sheath was performed (the distal angle of the sheath is not seen), there is almost 45 degrees angulation between the Amulet lobe and the sheath (panel **a**). As predicted by the MSCT, the Amulet lobe did not enter into the "wing". The position of the device is considered a bit proximal so a recapture (using the "triangular shape technique") and redeployment is performed resulting in a 2 mm deeper position. Again, the Amulet lobe does not fit in the "wing". The LAA ostium is denoted by the *green line*

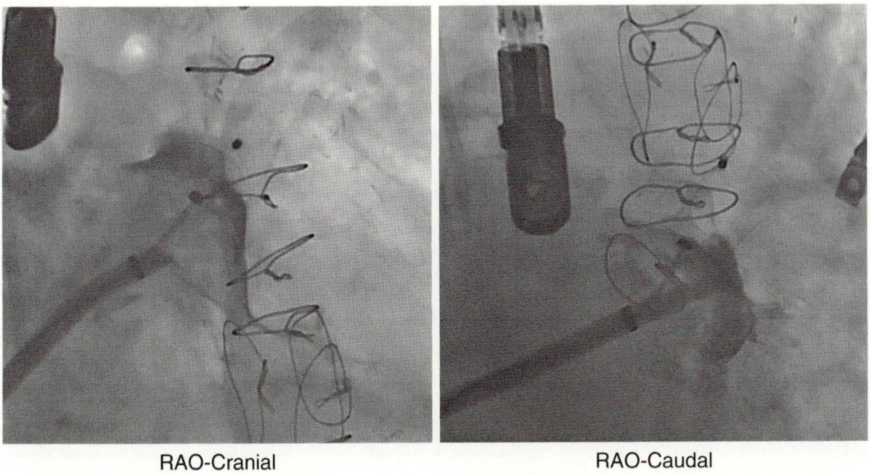

Fig. 8.20 Device evaluation by angiography in the RAO-Cranial and RAO-Caudal views shows complete LAA closure and good device position. All five signs of stability are present so after a short tug test the device is released. The was no peri-procedural complications and the follow-up TEE showed complete LAA closure without any leak

8.5 Cauliflower LAA with Short Depth

Learning objectives: How to deal with a short LAA depth in a patient with a cauliflower morphology.

TEE is a valuable tool to assess LAA diameters and morphology (Fig. 8.21). Similar to CT measurements, 3D TEE allows for the measurement of the LAA orifice and the device landing zone (Fig. 8.22) with good correlation to fluoroscopic measurements (Fig. 8.23). Similar to the above mentioned angio-guided procedures, the distal lobe of the Amulet is released in a triangular shape (Fig. 8.24). The proximal disc is released subsequently; a prolonged tug test is performed thereafter (Fig. 8.25). The final result shows a well-occluded LAA with the proximal disc covering the LAA in a typical concave shape (Figs. 8.26 and 8.27).

- In the case of a very oval LAA ostium/landing zone, the device can be chosen to be slightly smaller than the largest axial diameter.
- A careful pre-procedural evaluation is needed to ensure that the depth of the main anchoring lobe is sufficient to accomodate the selected device.
- Use of the triangular shape technique is helpful to implant the device safely deep into the LAA.
- To avoid the device popping out during the positioning of the lobe it can be helpful to gently push on the delivery cable.
- If suboptimal, pulling maneuvers may help to optimize the position of the disc.

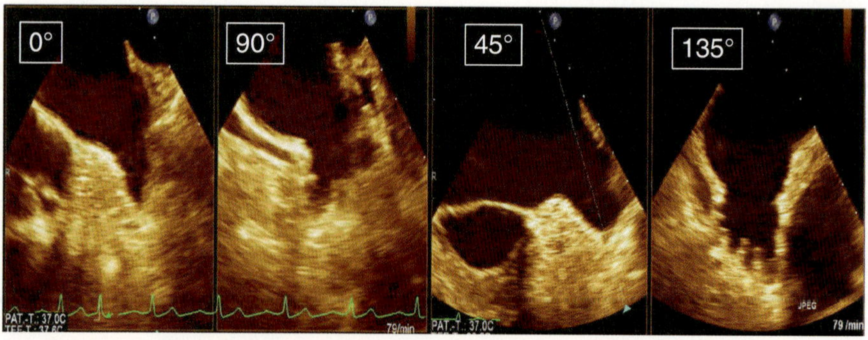

Fig. 8.21 The 2D TEE evaluation of the LAA in different planes reveals a cauliflower morphology with a short LAA depth (shortest measurement at 135° (see figure B)

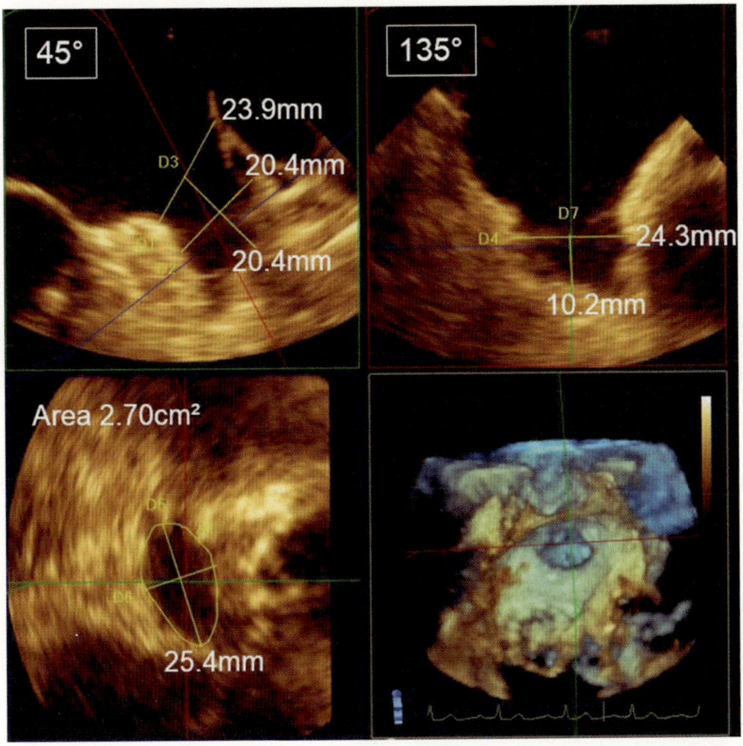

Fig. 8.22 The measurements of the ostium, the landing zone and the depth are shown in a 45 and a 135° view and in a 3D enface view (*bottom left*). The largest diameter is measured in the 3D enface view (25.4 mm). It can also be seen, that the shape of the LAA ostium is very eccentric and oval in shape. Derived from the area, a diameter of 19 mm is calculated. The depth is smallest in the 135° view (10.2 mm)

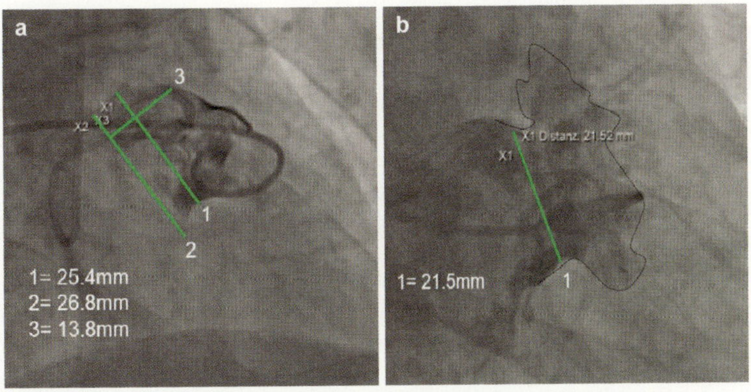

Fig. 8.23 Fluoroscopic measurements are shown ((**a**) RAO cranial and (**b**) RAO caudal): the largest diameter measured in fluoroscopy is also 25.4 mm. Due to the very eccentric shape of the LAA at the ostium and within the landing zone and an area derived diameter of only 19 mm, the device size is chosen slightly smaller than the largest diameter (25 mm Amulet)

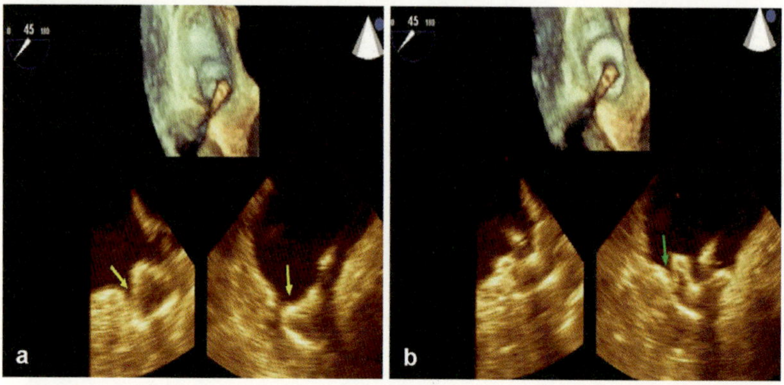

Fig. 8.24 The "triangular shape technique" ((**a**); *yellow arrows*) is used to safely develop the lobe of the Amulet device deep into this short LAA. The delivery cable is pushed gently to avoid a pop out of the lobe. (**b**) Assessment of the lobe shows a satisfactory position with good contact to the LAA wall in different imaging planes, particularly in the posterior region (*green arrow*). Therefore the disc can be developed in the next step

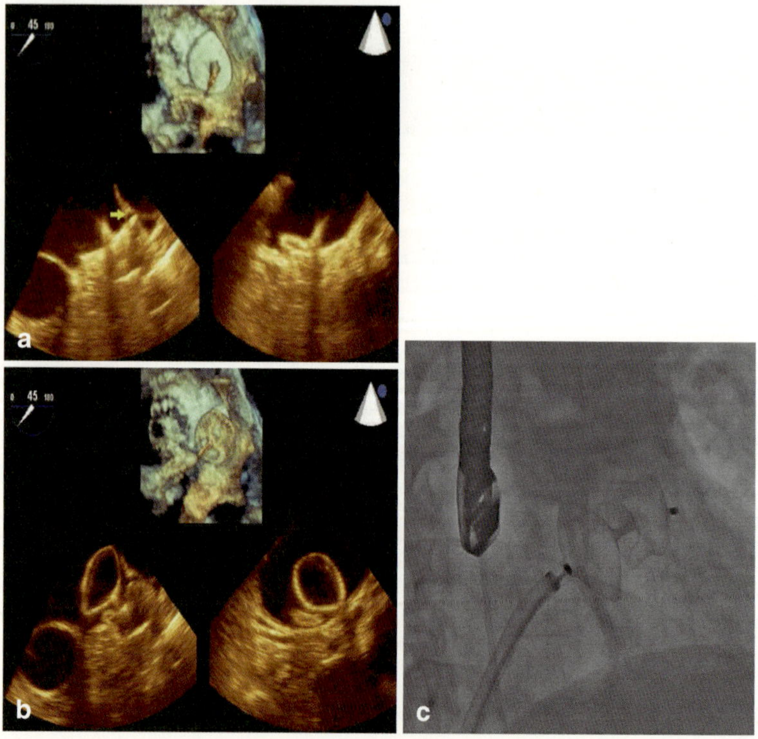

Fig. 8.25 The lateral part of the disc can be seen to be stuck in a small pouch of the lateral (cranial) LAA wall (*yellow arrow*) (**a**). Figures b and c: A prolonged tug test (approximately 2 min) is performed as shown in multiplanar TEE imaging (figure b) and on fluoroscopy (figure c) to confirm device stability and also to try to reposition the disc proximal to the small pouch

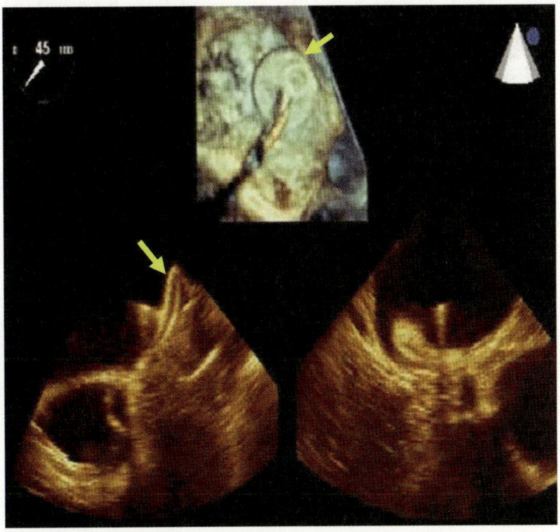

Fig. 8.26 Finally, after the tug test the disc covers the small pouch and adapts nicely to the lateral/cranial LAA wall (*yellow arrows*)

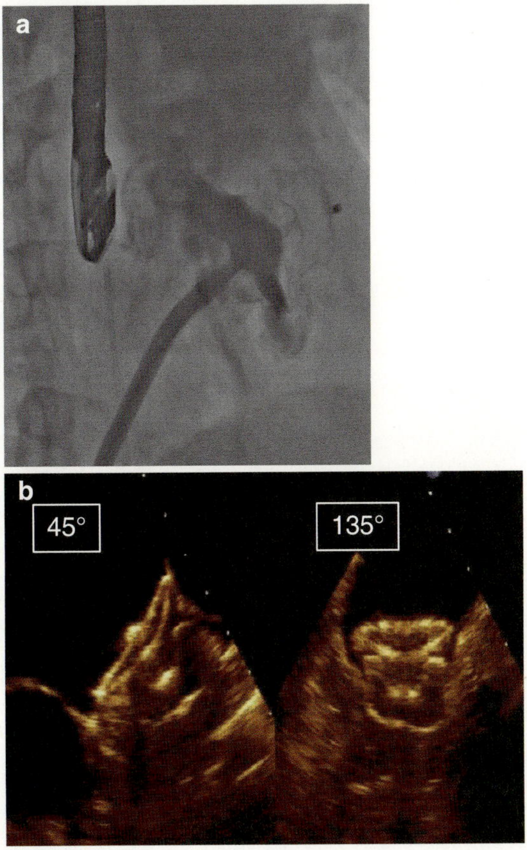

Fig. 8.27 The final angiogram with contrast injection confirms complete sealing of the LAA (**a**). The five signs of a stable device position are all fulfilled and the device is released. The final position of the 25 mm Amulet occluder is seen in a TEE X-plane view in figure b

8.6 LAA with a Chicken Wing Morphology and an Additional Proximal Lobe

Learning objectives: Decision making process in a patient with a formally unstable device position under tug test.

The initial echocardiographic images demonstrate a LAA with a chicken wing morphology with a late angulation (Fig. 8.28). Similar images are obtained by fluoroscopy (Fig. 8.29). The device is released from the sheath and engages the distal

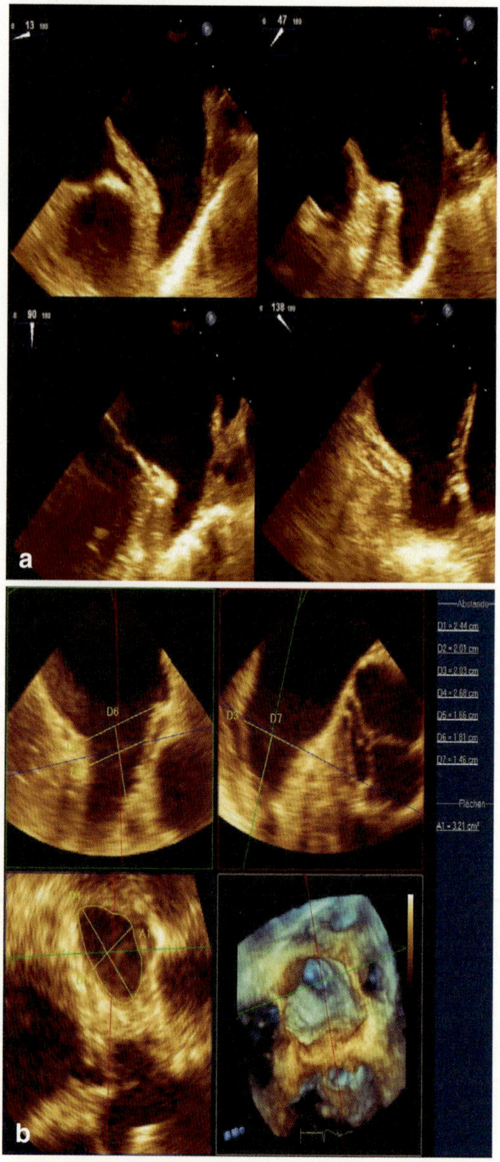

Fig. 8.28 (**a**) 2DTEE evaluation in different planes shows a chicken wing morphology with a late angulation and a good proximal landing zone. (**b**) The largest diameter is measured in the 3D enfac view (26.8 mm). The smallest diameter is 16.6 mm. The 3D enface view also demonstrates how oval this LAA ostium and the landing zone are

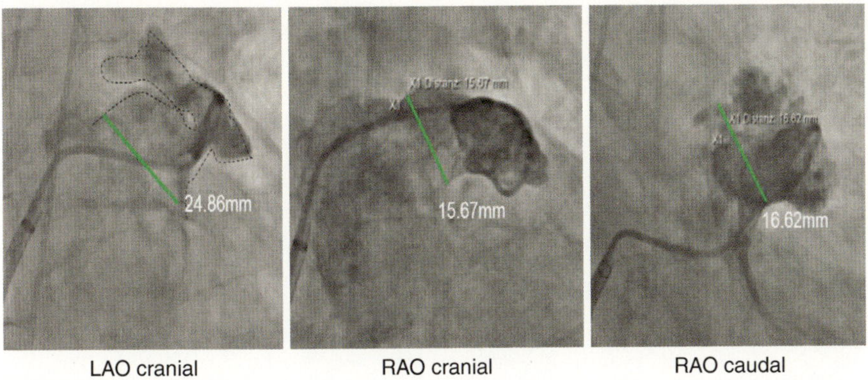

Fig. 8.29 Fluoroscopic images confirm the chicken wing morphology and the eccentricity of the LAA ostium

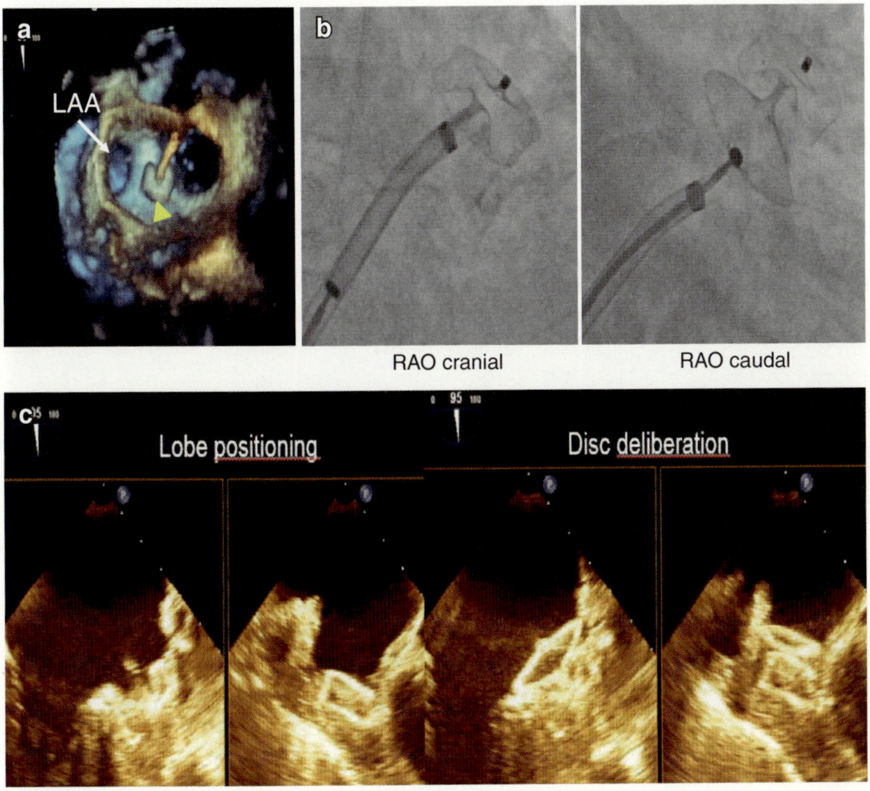

Fig. 8.30 (**a**) The "ball technique" is used as seen in a 3D enface view. The "ball" (*yellow arrowhead*) is directed towards the LAA entrance. The positioning of the lobe and the deployment of the disc is shown fluoroscopically (**b**) and in X-plane TEE views (**c**)

LAA employing the "ball technique" (Fig. 8.30). The tug test finds the superior part of the device moving (Fig. 8.31). An additional lobe was overlooked on the initial TEE (Fig. 8.32). A prolonged tug tests finds the device to be stable despite protruding into the LA at the superior border (Fig. 8.33). The device is relased and confirmed to fully occlude the LAA (Fig. 8.34).

- All five release criteria should be fulfilled before a device is unscrewed.
- In the case of an unstable device position, the exact mechanism has to be defined.

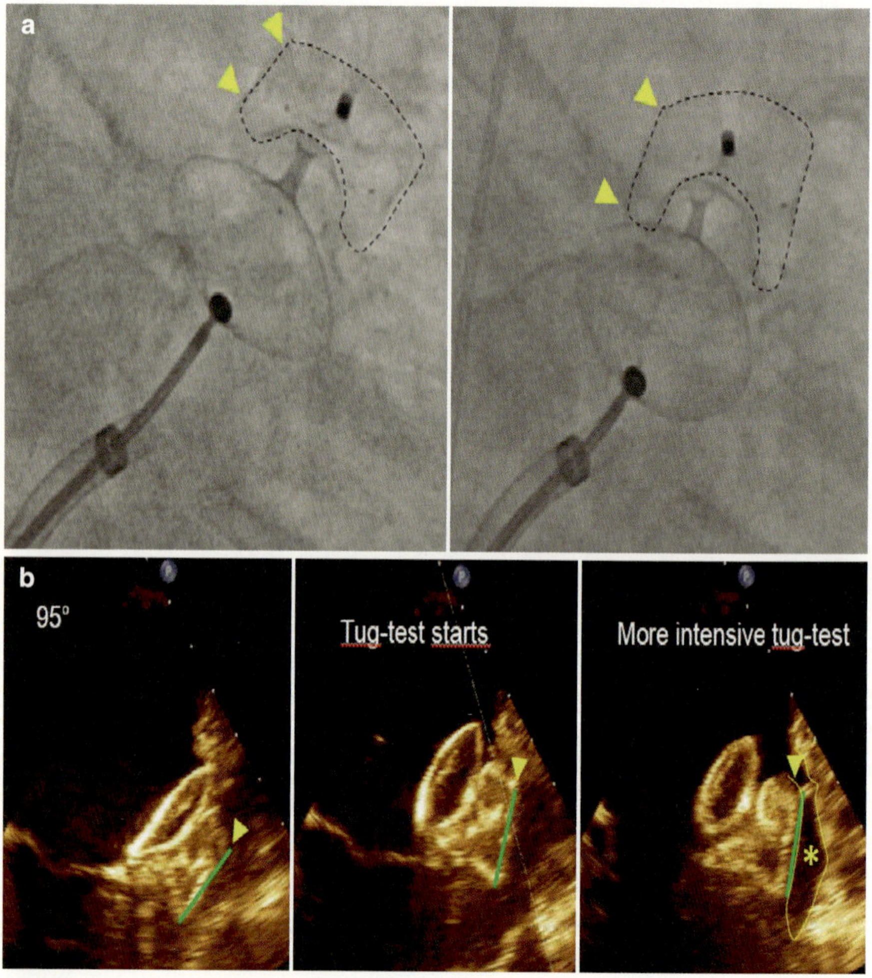

Fig. 8.31 (**a**) Four of the release criteria are fulfilled, but under tug test a relevant movement of the device at the lateral wall (cranial) can be observed (*yellow arrowheads*) in fluoroscopy. The tug test as seen in TEE images (**b**) reveals that the lobe of the device is not attached to the lateral wall of the LAA but to a very floppy tissue bridge in between the main anchoring lobe and a proximal lateral side lobe (marked with a yellow asterisk) (this side lobe has not been seen in fluoroscopy or TEE so far). The caudal part of the device is stable during the tug test

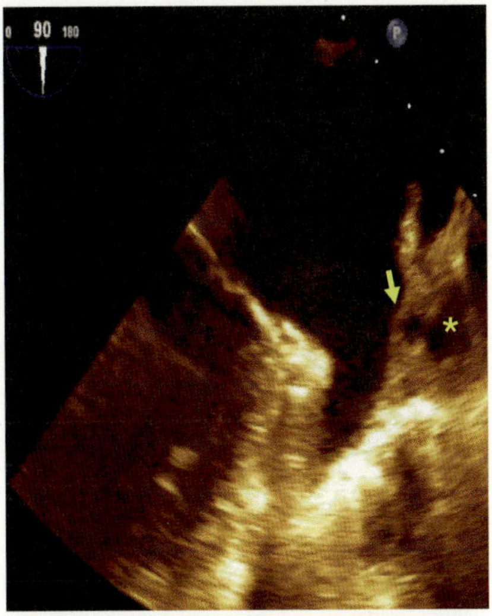

Fig. 8.32 Retrospectively the side lobe (*yellow asterisk*) can be identified in the 90° view. The entrance is covered by tissue (*yellow arrow*)

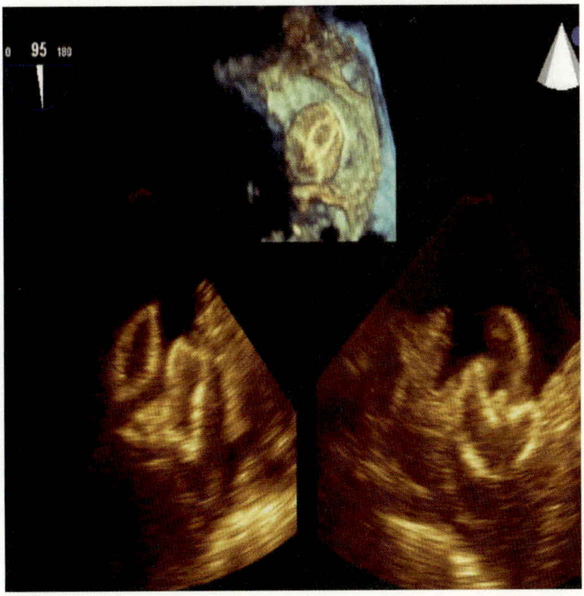

Fig. 8.33 Multiple prolonged tug tests are performed and confirm that the device is safely attached to the mobile tissue bridge

- Different imaging modalities may be helpful. In this case the mechanism was clarified by the use of TEE.

In this case the device seemed to be unstable, but the attachment of the device to the mobile tissue bridge in between the main anchoring lobe and a lateral side lobe was stable and the side lobe was adequately sealed during the normal cardiac cycle. Therefore the tug test was finally judged to be positive and the device was released.

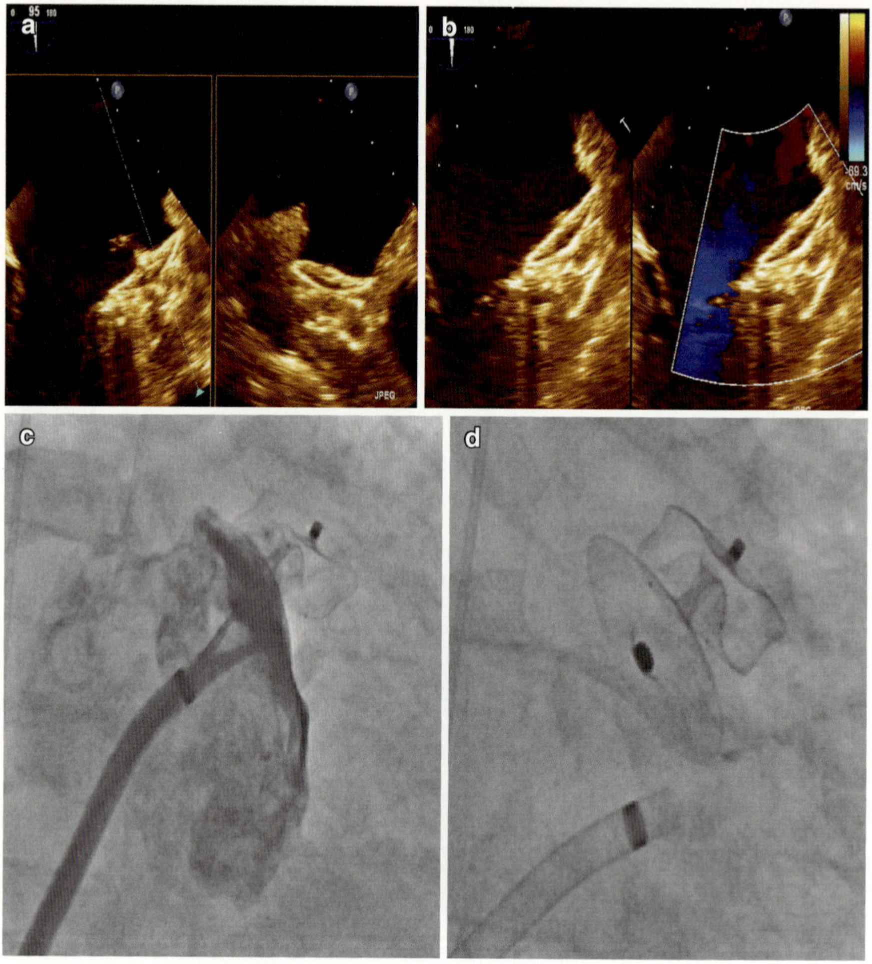

Fig. 8.34 After each tug test the device comes always back to the same unchanged position (**a**) and no color flow around the device is detectable (**b**). This confirms that the disc covers the side lobe adequately. This finding is also confirmed fluoroscopically with contrast injection (**c**). Therefore the decision is made that the device is stable and it is released uneventfully (**d**)

8.7 Closing a LAA with a Close Proximity to the Pulmonary Artery

Learning objective: evaluation of surrounding structures is important for LAA closure using the Amulet device.

This particular LAA looks "innocent" at first glance; it is a single lobe LAA with a windsock shape (Fig. 8.35). Yet a slightly different TEE angle (10°) shows the pulmonary artery to be very close to the landing zone of the Amulet in the LAA

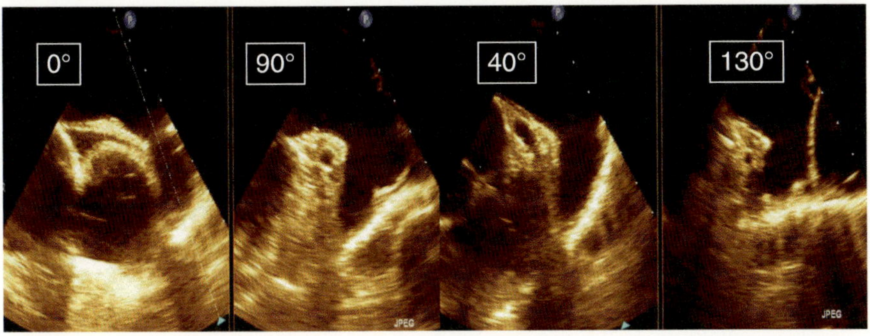

Fig. 8.35 TEE in different imaging planes shows a single lobe LAA with a windsock shape

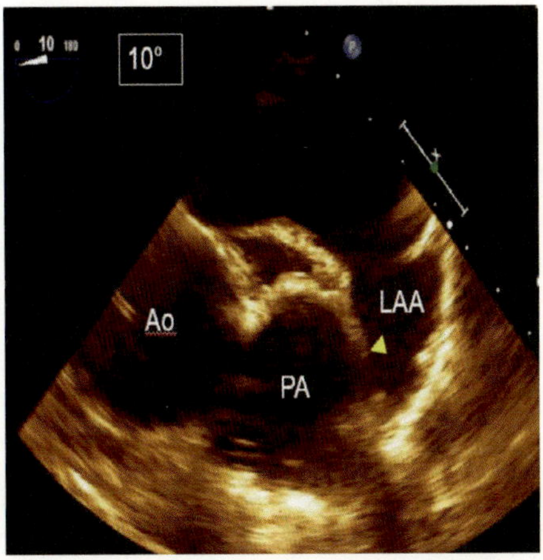

Fig. 8.36 A closer look at this 10° TEE view shows that the pulmonary artery (PA) is positioned between the left atrial appendage (LAA) and the aorta (Ao). The *yellow arrowhead points* out how thin the tissue layers between the LAA wall and the pulmonary artery are. The risk of device perforation into the pulmonary artery is therefore increased

(Fig. 8.36). As a strategy to avoid potential perforation of the device anchors into the pulmonary artery, the distal lobe is sized in a manner that allows for the device to be positioned obliquely (Fig. 8.37). Angiographic measurements confirm this placement (Fig. 8.38). Device release is performed under fluoroscopic guidance (Fig. 8.39). TEE confirms this initial strategy has worked (Fig. 8.40). The final tug test confirms correct sizing and anchoring of the device (Fig. 8.41).

- A pulmonary artery underlying the LAA can result in a very close anatomical relationship with an increased risk of perforation.
- The evaluation of surrounding structures and the relationship to each other is therefore of major importance and may influence implantation strategies.
- TEE or alternatively CT imaging adds additional information to fluoroscopic imaging in the evaluation of surrounding structures.

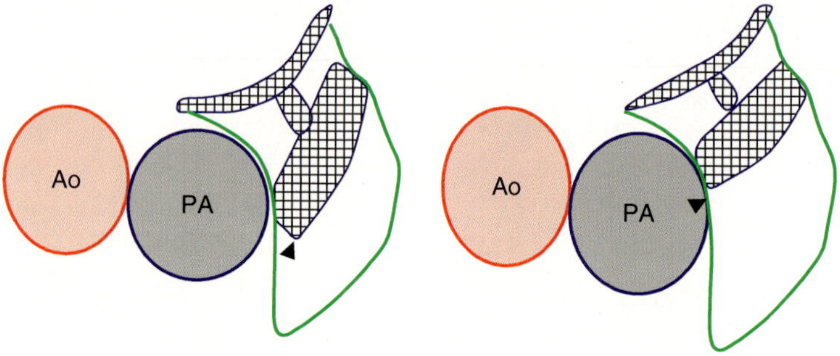

Fig. 8.37 To minimize the risk of perforation a strategy was planned to chose a larger device size and to implant the lobe more obliquely as demonstrated on the left side to keep the hooks (*black arrow*) away from the pulmonary artery rather than implanting a smaller device in a conventional position as seen on the right side with the hooks (*black arrow*) pointing directly towards the pulmonary artery

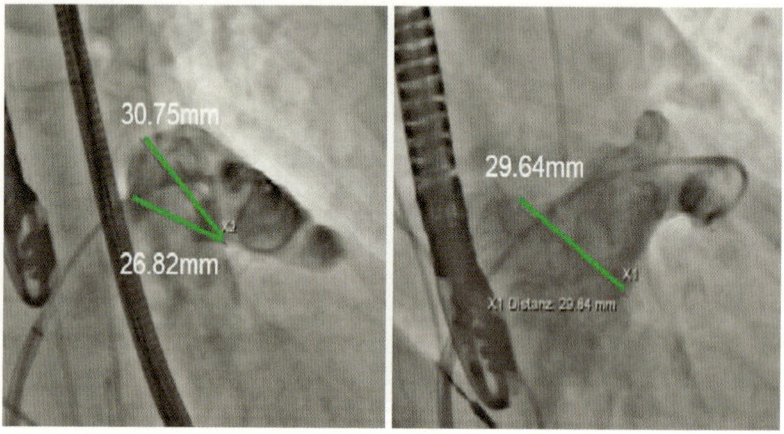

Fig. 8.38 Fluoroscopic images confirm the windsock type LAA. Measurements are performed according to the planned implantation strategy

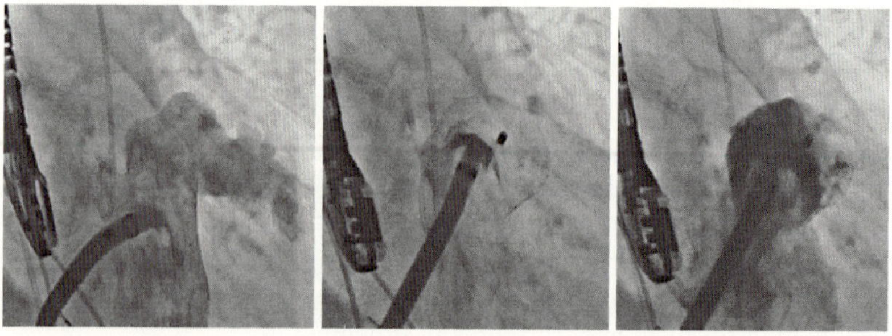

Fig. 8.39 The positioning of the lobe is demonstrated fluoroscopically in a RAO caudal projection. Contrast injections confirm no flow into the distal LAA cavity

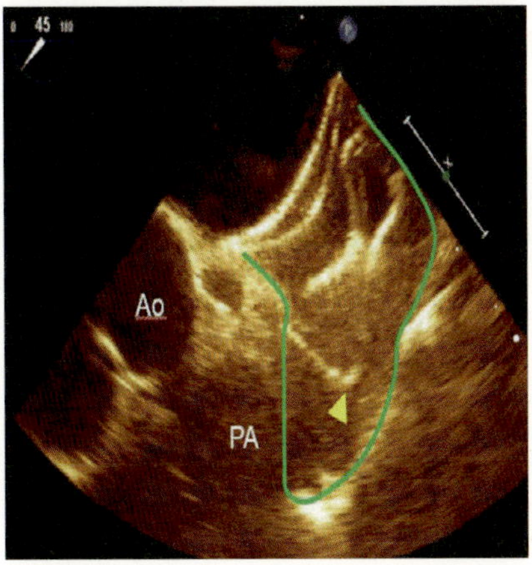

Fig. 8.40 The final device position is seen in a 45° TEE view. The hooks (*yellow arrowhead*) are pointing to the free lumen of the distal LAA cavity and not towards the pulmonary artery

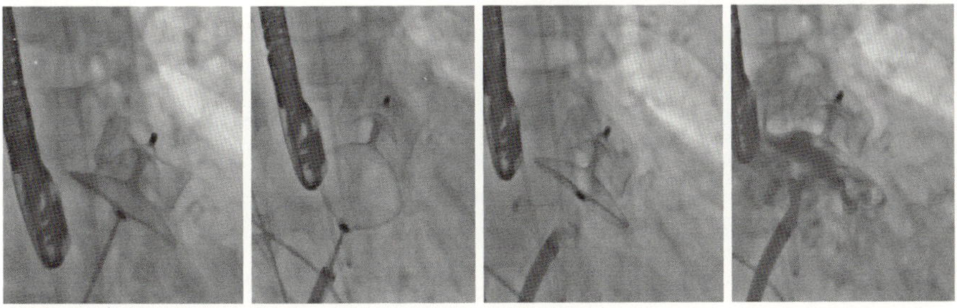

Fig. 8.41 The final shape of the device after the positioning of the disc is seen (*leftmost*). A stable device position is confirmed by a tug test (*middle left*). After device release (*middle right*) the position is unchanged and a final angiogram confirms complete sealing of the LAA (*rightmost*)

Acknowledgment The author would like to thank Kevin P. Walsh, Mater Misericordiae University Hospital, Dublin, Ireland for critical reading and helpful comments.

Chapter 9
Prevention and Management of Complications

9.1 Procedure

9.1.1 Pericardial Effusion/Tamponade

Pericardial effusion/tamponade is probably the most common complication of LAA closure (Fig. 9.1, panel a). Careful step-by-step LAA closure technique has decreased initial pericardial effusion rates of around 5% down to less than 1%. Perforation of the LAA, the left atrial wall or (rarely) the pulmonary vein can occur at anytime during the procedure (during transseptal puncture, stiff wire introduction, sheath exchange, device deployment, etc.), (Fig. 9.1, panel b). According to the latest Munich consensus definitions, and based on the time it occurs, pericardial effusion/tamponade is categorized as intraprocedural, acute (≤48 h from the index procedure) or late (>48 h from the index procedure) [7].

9.1.1.1 Prevention

- By using TEE, the baseline status of pericardial space should be defined in order to differentiate an acute from chronic pericardial effusion.
- Optionally, two packs of RBC may be cross-matched before the procedure.
- LAA closure in a patient receiving OAC therapy should be avoided.
- During transseptal puncture, all available safety measures should be used, especially when encountering a very rigid or aneurysmal interatrial septum. For example, a coronary angioplasty wire can be used. The stiff back-end of the wire is used to puncture (insidc the TSP needle—not to be advanced more then 3–5 mm in the left atrium) and then the floppy front of the wire can be advanced in the left upper pulmonary vein (LSPV) to facilitate safe introduction of the TSP sheath (over-the-wire). In case of a rigid septum, the dilator and sheath can be advanced over the introducer wire (0.032″) that has been carefully placed in the LSPV.

M.W. Bergmann et al., *Clinical Cases in LAA Occlusion*,
DOI 10.1007/978-3-319-51431-4_9

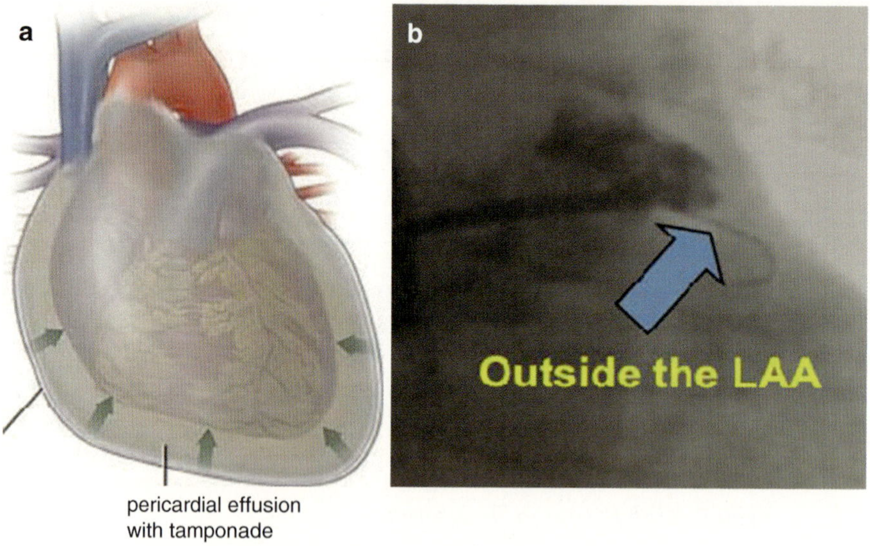

Fig. 9.1 (**a**) Pericardial effusion and cardiac tamponade is the most common complication of LAA closure. (**b**) The LAA is a delicate cardiac structure that can be easily perforated. Any wire (even a J wire) that is pushed out of a catheter can perforate the LAA if the catheter is against the LAA wall. Unsheathing and fluoroscopic guidance is recommended. The SafeSept wire can be used for a safer transseptal puncture

- Angiography of the LAA should be performed via a pigtail catheter (inside the TSP sheath) or via the side arm of the TSP sheath. The latter allows for enhanced contrast injection in high pressure, which can fully dilate a partially collapsed LAA (especially a large LAA). Power injection should be avoided and checking for back-flow bleeding before injecting can prevent LAA wall trauma from a vigorous contrast injection.
- Since the LAA is a blind-ended structure, any wire should be advanced cautiously and only under fluoroscopic guidance. Note that even a soft J wire can easily perforate the LAA when it is pushed out a catheter facing the LAA wall (Fig. 9.1, panel b).
- Early detection of a pericardial effusion can be life saving so close patient monitoring is required. An invasive pressure line (i.e. radial) can allow for immediate recognition of hemodynamic compromise due to pericardial effusion. The TEE operator should check periodically for the presence of a new effusion.
- When deep intubation of the LAA is needed a pigtail catheter should be used inside the TSP or the delivery sheath.
- A pericardial drainage kit should be readily available in the Cath Lab.
- When available, a cardiac surgeon should be notified about a planned LAA closure procedure.
- Watchman implantation: a very distal release in a tiny lobe (Fig. 9.2) where the device cannot unfold properly also leaving a large gap (Fig. 9.2b, c, d) has a high risk of causing a pericardial effusion.

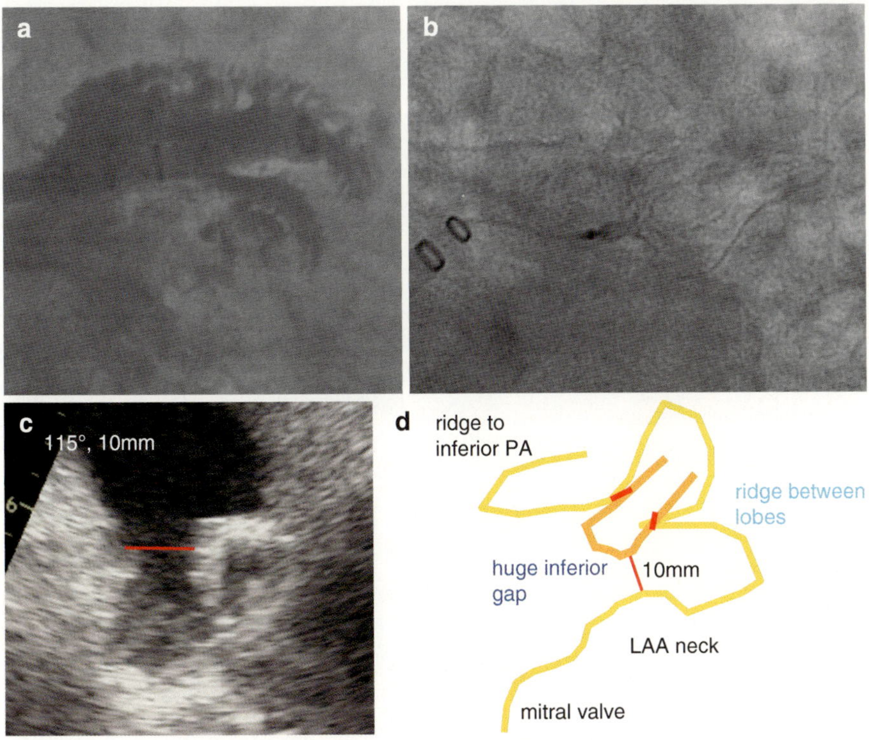

Fig. 9.2 *Pericardial effusion following distal release* (**a**) The Watchman delivery sheath is positioned deep in the most anterior lobe. The 27 mm device is released (**b**) but leaves a huge gap towards the inferior lobe (**c**, **d**). The ridge between the lobes which is not visible on TEE (see Fig. 8.1) prevents the device taking the typical Watchman configuration. The device is compressed massively in its distal part (**b**). This situation (device release too distal, compression >70%) comes with a particular high risk of pericardial effusion

9.1.1.2 Treatment

A rapidly accumulating pericardial effusion is an emergency situation because it can lead to tamponade and cardiac arrest within a few minutes. The following measures should be applied.

- If the device is closing the LAA effectively, it should be released since this will minimize leakage from the LAA (Fig. 9.3).
- LAA closure should be completed rapidly if possible. Successful LAA closure either with an Amplatzer Amulet or a Watchman device will often seal or at least partially seal the source of hemorrhage.
- echo diagnosis should be made by comparing baseline images to the current situation (Fig. 9.4a, b).
- Pericardiocentesis should be performed once the effusion has reached approximately 1 cm (Fig. 9.4b). Puncture is easily performed with a standard long

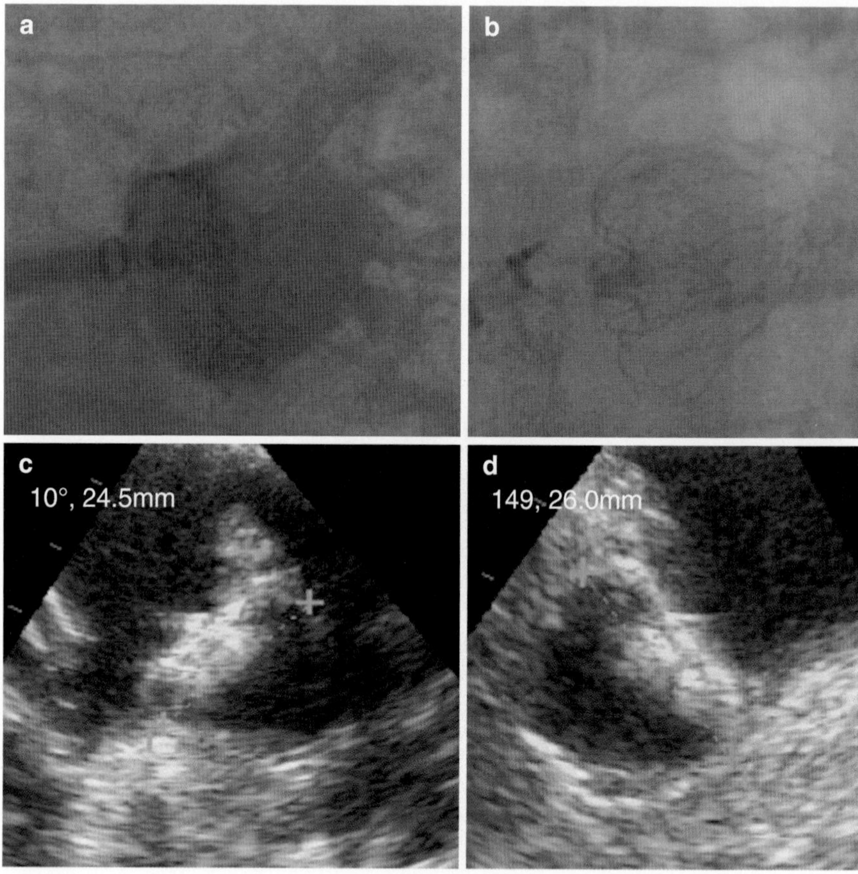

Fig. 9.3 *Successful closure of the LAA with a more proximal release*. After partial recapture the device is release more proximal finally taking the classical Watchman strawberry-like configuration (**a**, **b**). Echo confirms good compression and successful closure without any leaks (**c**, **d**)

needle from a pericardial puncture set with small amounts of contrast medium to visualize successful location of the epicardial space. (Fig. 9.4c) Very early puncture has an increased risk of accidental right ventricular puncture. Late puncture takes the risk of the patient becoming hemodynamically stable.

- 6F Pigtail via a standard femoral sheath is recommended. (Fig. 9.4d)
- Ongoing hemorrhage may be managed by autotransfusion using a standard red blood cell transfusion system and a 50 ml syringe
- Reversal of heparinization with protamine risks thrombus formation in the epicardial space without stopping bleeding; the pigtail clots but the effusion continues to enlarge. This regularly ends in a very unstable situation which requires immediate surgery and is responsible for the mortality in this setting. Usually the bleeding reduces after around 10–15 min of drainage even without protamin.

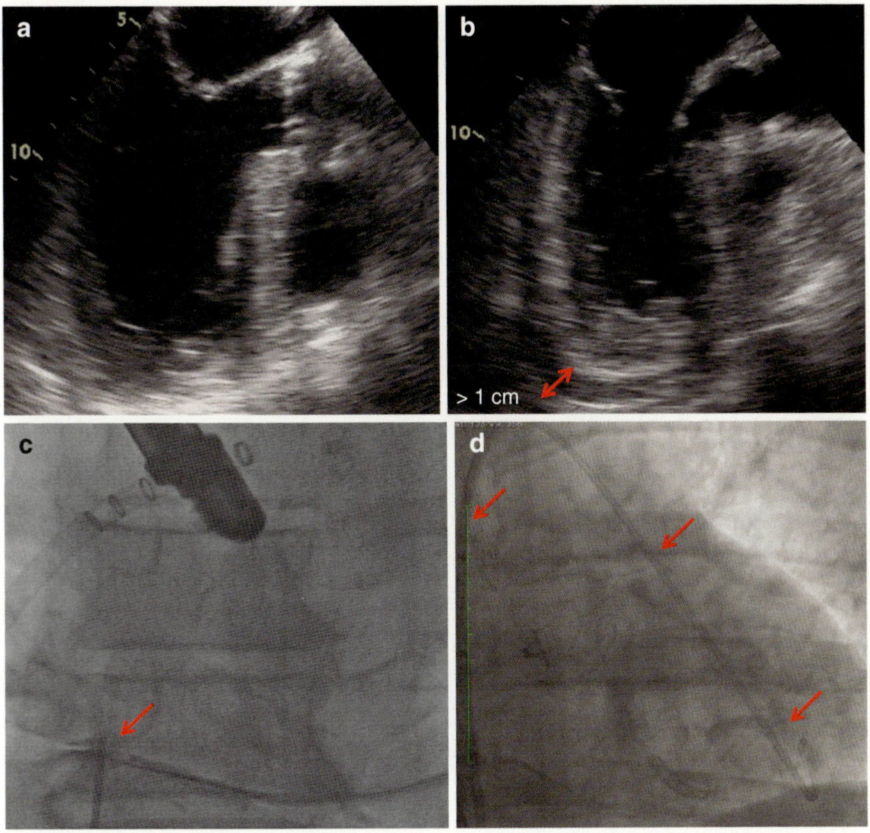

Fig. 9.4 *Pericardial effusion following the first distal Watchman release; successful drainage.* Parallel to LAA closure demonstrated in Figs. 8.1–8.3 the development of a hemodynamically relevant pericardial effusion is observed (**a**, **b**). A pericardial puncture under angiographic guidance is performed from a subxiphoid access (**c**) using contrast to visualize correct positioning of the needle. A 6F pigtail is placed in the pericardial space (**d**). This drained around 200 cc of blood. No protamine is given since this would lead to clotting of the pericardial effusion without sealing the perfoaration resulting in impaired effective pericardial drainage.

- In case of massive hemorrhage, call for emergency surgery preparation.
- Most pericardial effusion's can be managed by interventional pericardiocentesis. Usually drainage is required for around 24–48 h.

9.1.2 Thrombus Formation

Thrombus formation during LAA closure can occur within seconds and can jeopardize the whole procedure. Incomplete heparinization is the most common reason for thrombus formation (Fig. 9.5).

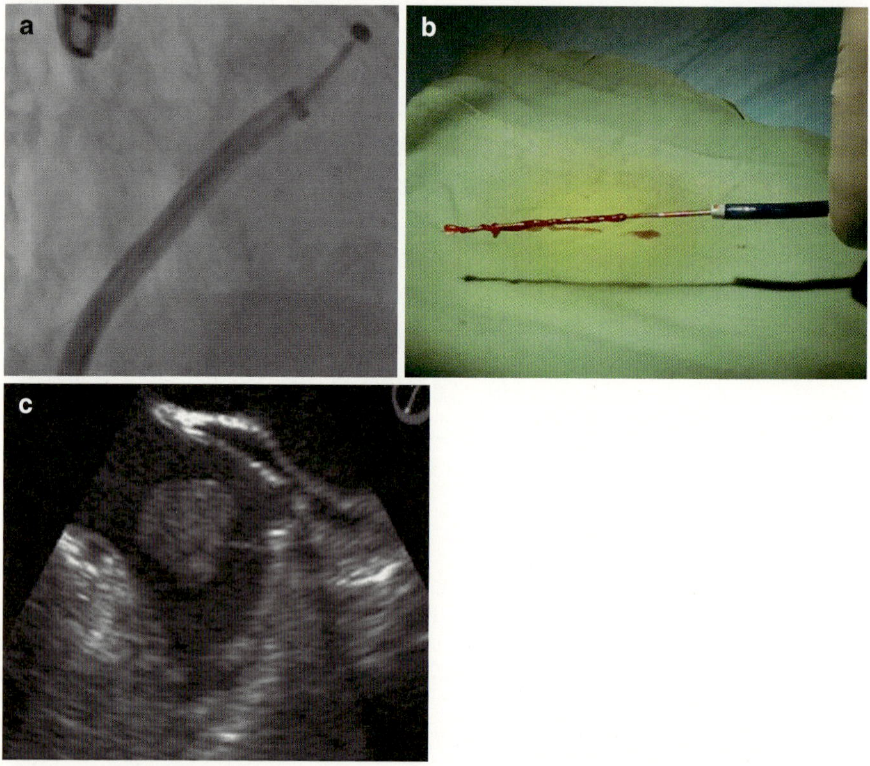

Fig. 9.5 (**a**) Thrombus is not visible on fluoroscopy unless contrast is injected. However, as this may result in thrombus embolization to the periphery it should be avoided. (**b**) Fortunately, to date delivery wire thrombosis has not been associated with procedural stroke as the thrombotic material is attached quite firmly to the wire. In any case, careful heparinization with an ACT > 250 s (or even 300 s) is mandatory. (**c**) TEE surveillance is invaluable in the early detection of thrombus in the LAA, on the LAA closure device or delivery system

9.1.2.1 Prevention

- ACT should be periodically checked (every 20–30 min) and corrected.
- ACT should be between 250–300 sec before introducing any material in the left atrium.
- In the case of a difficult TSP, a thrombus can form on the TSP needle in the right atrium. Therefore many operators prefer to administer half-dose of heparin before TSP and complete heparinization immediately after crossing the septum.
- Some patients may have a higher risk for thrombosis due to very large left atria, chronic AF with spontaneous contrast on TEE, blood dyscrasias or resistance to heparin and, therefore, require higher doses of heparin. On the other hand, there is always a theoretical risk of bleeding, which is commonly the indication for LAA closure, so aggressive heparinization may be harmful. Time is probably

one of the most important elements: if working on a low ACT range is mandatory, the intervention should be done as speedily as possible.
- Thrombus is usually not visible on fluoroscopy so TEE surveillance is important for early detection.
- For the Amplatzer devices, the most common surface a thrombus may be formed on is the distal part of the delivery wire. Fortunately, when a thrombus forms there it is well attached and does not easily embolize to the periphery.
- If the patient is not sufficiently heparinized, thrombus may develop inside the Watchman sheath. If after the transseptal puncture and sheath exchange, backbleeding is unsuccessful, the sheath should be removed and flushed outside the body.

9.1.2.2 Treatment

- Depending on its position, size and mobility, thrombus aspiration via a large sheath may be attempted.
- Local thrombolysis with alteplase has been reported.
- If available, it is advisable to use a cerebral protection device before starting any manipulations.
- The presence of thrombus in the LAA despite adequate OAC (Fig. 9.6a) is a challenging situation (malignant LAA). At first presentation, the patient should be treated with low molecular weight heparin for 4–6 weeks.
- If the thrombus persists, LAA closure may be discussed. Several procedures have been performed without sequelae. The use of a cerebral protection device like the Claret device (Sentinel; used in transcatheter aortic valve implantation (TAVI) procedures) is recommended (Figs. 9.6, 9.7 and 9.8).
- A Watchman device can be implanted proximal to the thrombus; this implantation should be done without visualizing the depth of the LAA with contract injection.

9.1.3 Device Embolization

Device embolization can occur in almost any interventional cardiology procedure. The anatomical variability of the LAA (particularly shallow, cone shaped configurations) may increase the risk for device embolization (Fig. 9.9).

9.1.3.1 Prevention

- Release of the device only if tug test and device conformation fulfills the release criteria
- Use of TEE is mandatory. Cardiac CT is a valuable tool for understanding the anatomy ahead of the implant procedure.

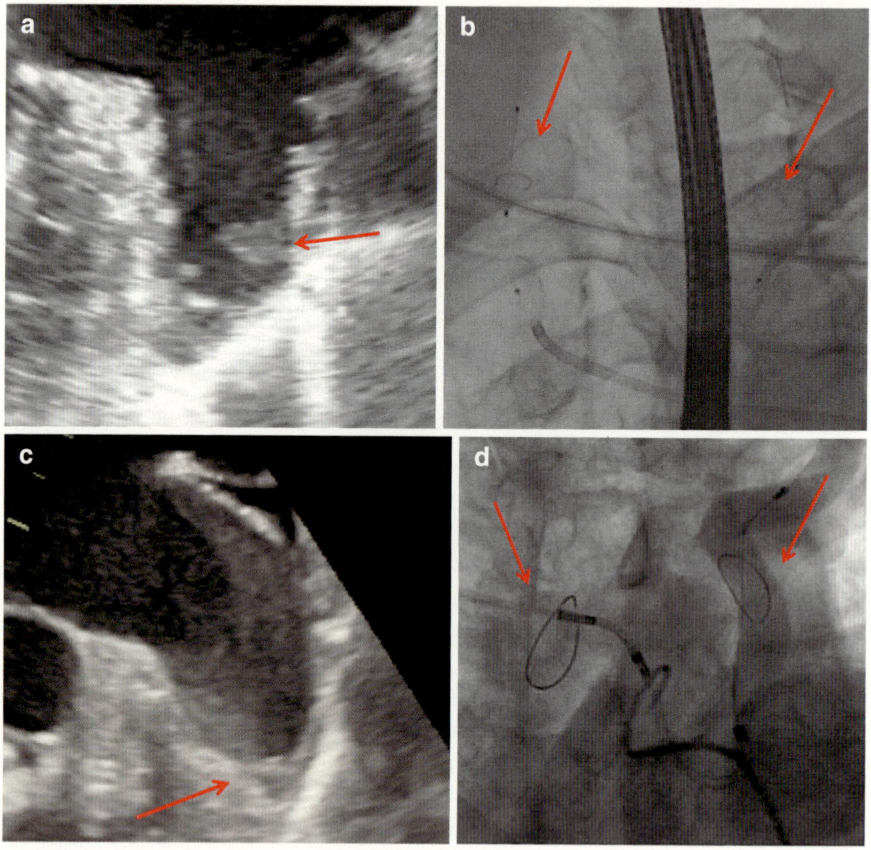

Fig. 9.6 *LAA closure in the presence of thrombus*. Two patients are shown with clear thrombus (**a**, *red arrow*) or massive sludge with unclear delineation of LAA trabeculation but possible distal thrombus (**b**, *red arrow*)) despite full oral anticoagulation >4 weeks with either low molecular weight heparin (patient 1 **a**, **c**) or INR >2.5 (patient 2, **c**, **d**). Carotid protection devices (**b**: Spider FX embolic protection device, Ev3) **c**: Sentinel carotid protection device, Claret Medical) were placed prior to transseptal puncture and LAA closure. Neither of the two patients had an event or detectable thrombus in the protection device after removal

- Correct device sizing; if in doubt i.e. for Watchman sizing use the larger device
- Checking the connection between the device and the delivery wire before pushing the device out of the sheath.
- After device deployment, use the stability checkpoints and tests according to the instruction for use.
- Awareness of imaging limitations. A 2-dimensional technique like fluoroscopy or 2D TEE may miss important information regarding device stability and apposition. Therefore, it is recommended to use more than one view for device assessment.

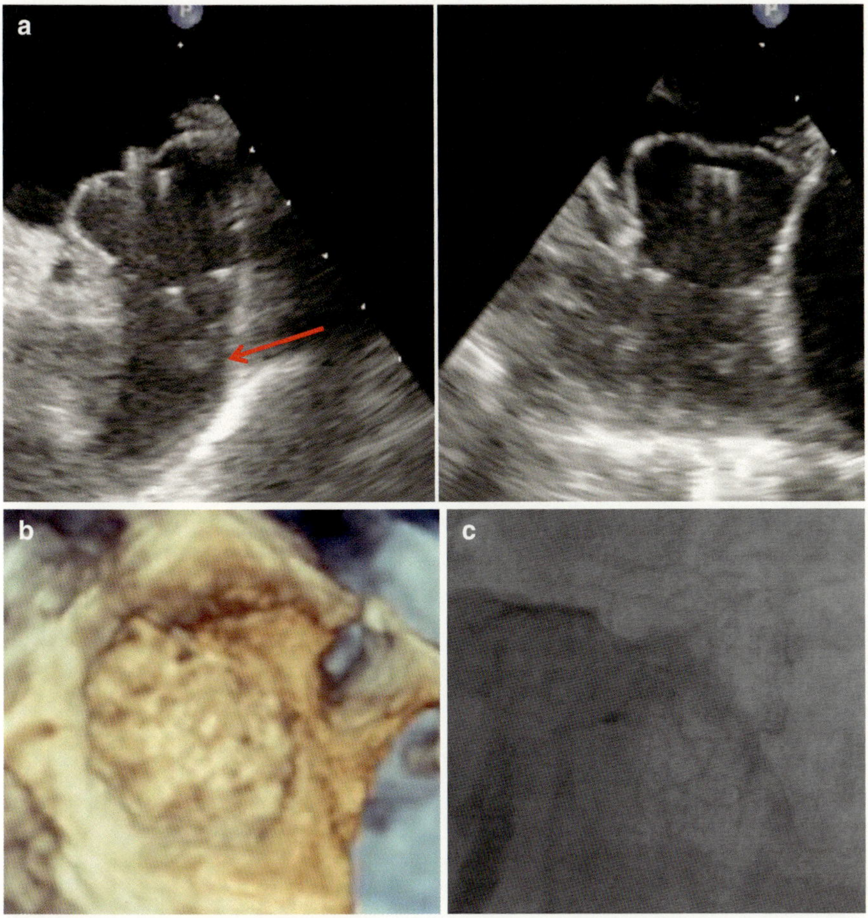

Fig. 9.7 *Echo-guided LAA closure in the presence of thrombus*. For a patient with mobile thrombus (Fig. 8.5, **a**, **b**) the Watchman procedure can be performed with good results with only echo guidance. The 30 mm Watchman was deployed in the classical landing zone without the pigtail being used to negotiate the depth of the LAA. Successfull closure of the LAA (**a**–**c**) with the thrombus still visible distal to the Watchman (*red arrow*) was achieved

- Waiting for a few minutes after device deployment and before release (i.e. 10–15′) may allow the device to settle better and find its final position. This is particularly important for the two part Amulet device.
- Always reassess the device position and signs of stability after a tug test has been performed. Using stored fluoroscopy/angiography as a reference point can help identify minor device displacements.
- Extra caution is needed when using a large ACP or Amulet device (i.e. > 25 mm) because after migration it will probably remain in the left atrium or move to the left ventricle, where it is more difficult to snare.
- Most embolizations occur early so surveillance during the first 24 h is required.

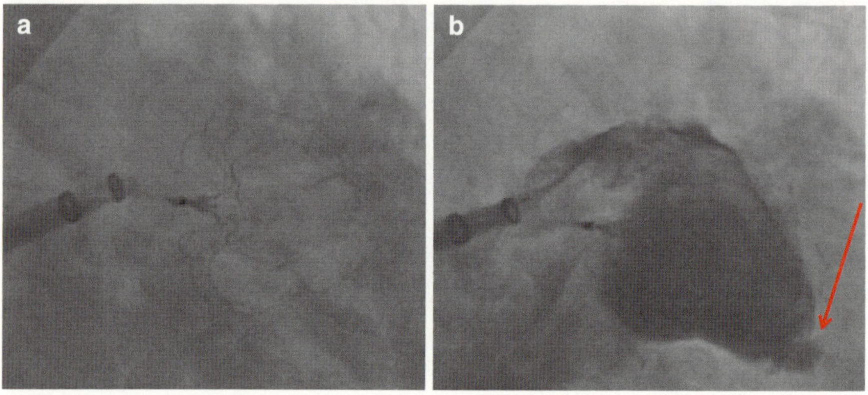

Fig. 9.8 *LAA closure in the presence of thrombus*. For patient 2 (sludge, possible distal thrombus) routine LAA closure was performed with the device spanning the proximal landing zone (**a**, **b**). One may speculate whether angiography (contrast can move through the PET fabric of the Watchman mesh, yet no thrombus will be able to leave the LAA through the device) visualizes the distal thrombus or whether this is trabeculated LAA tissue (*red arrow*)

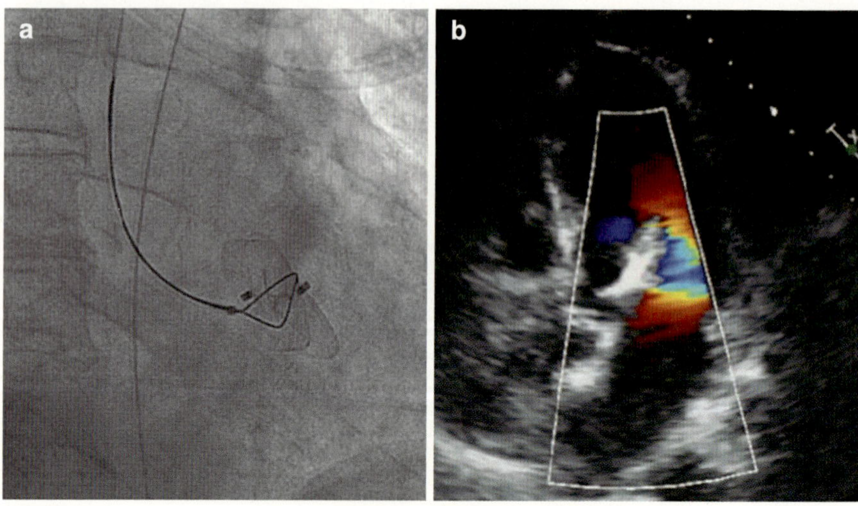

Fig. 9.9 An embolized Amplatzer Cardiac Plug or Amulet device can be snared in the left atrium, the left ventricle, in the aorta or the iliac arteries. If the device embolizes in the right heart circulation it can be snared in the pulmonary arteries. Fig. a–d demonstrate the space

9.1.3.2 Treatment

- In the majority of cases the embolized device can be removed percutaneously using retrieval devices like snares, bioptomes, etc., femoral access through the common femoral artery and a large TAVI sheath. A 16F sheath (i.e. from Cook)

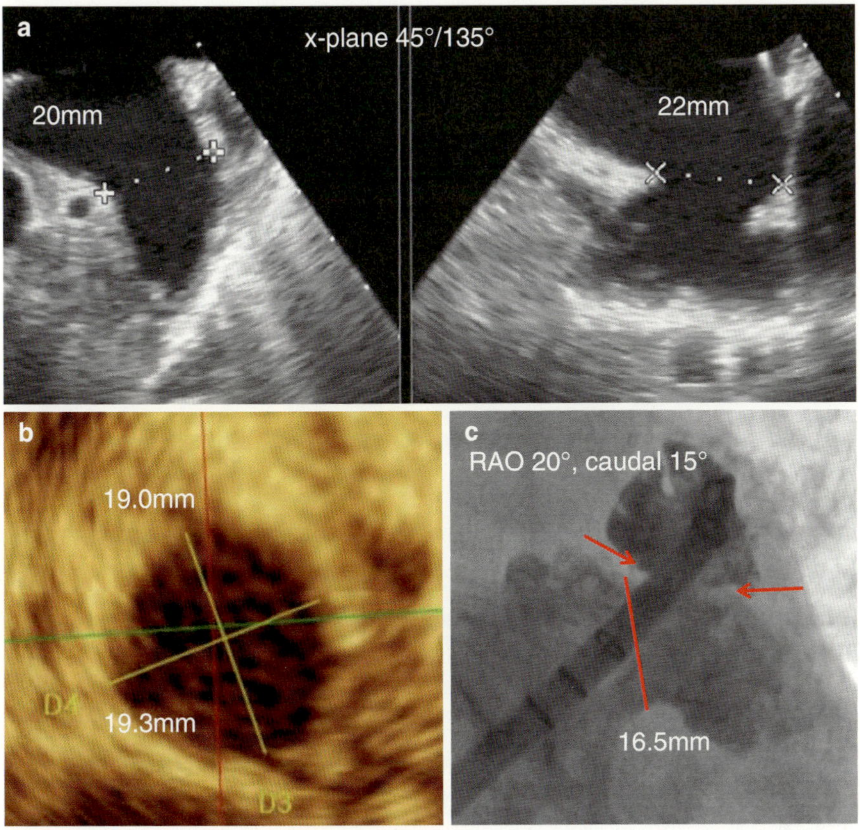

Fig. 9.10 *Watchman device embolization*. Challenging anatomy with two lobes and a small tubular entrance (*arrows, 9.10 a+b*) to the preferred landing zone in the anterior lobe (**c**). A 24 mm Watchman device was selected after the measurements were taken

should be available. It is advisable to have different types of snares available in the Cath Lab, together with large sheaths of different length.

- Snaring an LAA closure device may be extremely challenging. Several tricks may be applied depending on the device type, position, mobility and size. As a general rule one should avoid major entanglement with the mitral valve because it can be easily damaged.
- The Watchman device usually embolizes to the inferior aorta (Figs. 9.10, 9.11 and 9.12). A 16F TAVI sheath may be used for removal after snaring the device employing a large loop snare. As an alternative, a stiff wire (i.e. Supracore 260 cm) may be used to first advance the wire through the metal cage of the device and then snare the wire proximal to the device. Device, snare and wire may then be retracted through a 16F sheath.
- LAA may be closed with the same type of device but with a larger diameter following successful snaring of the device (Fig. 9.13)

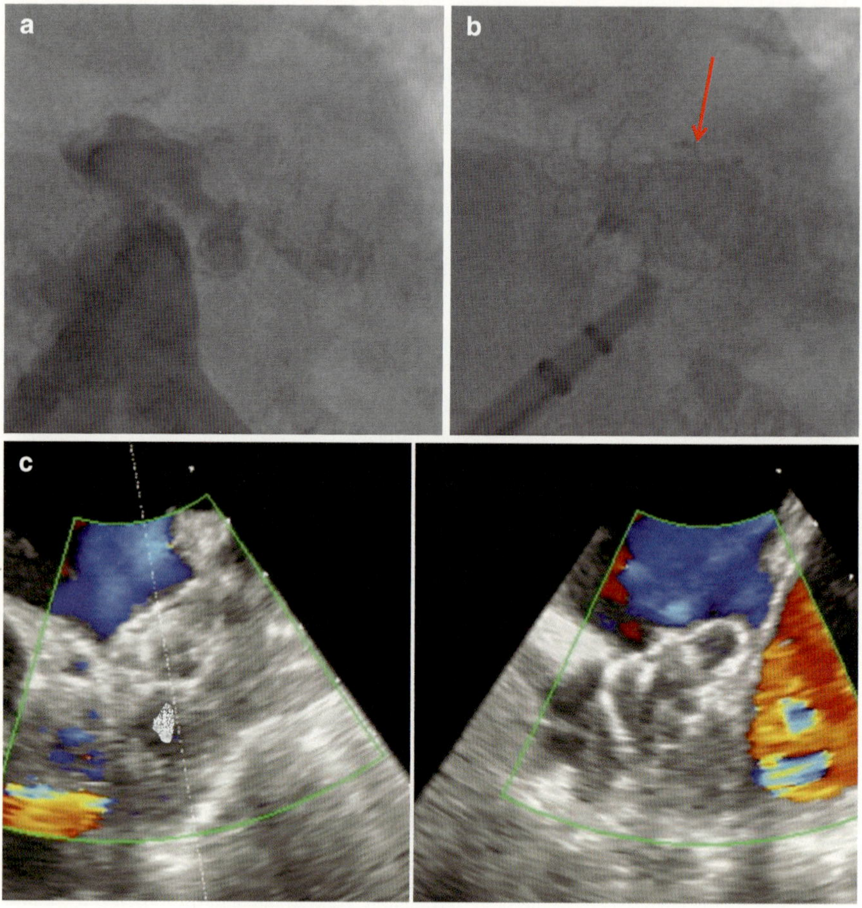

Fig. 9.11 *Watchman device embolization*. The 24 mm Watchman takes on a strange conformation (**b**, **c**), however tug test, sealing and compression is positive (**a**, images not shown). The device is therefore released in the position demonstrated

9.1.4 Air Embolism

Air embolism is a rare complication of LAA closure and it usually caused by poor operator technique (Fig. 9.14). Introduction of air in the left heart circulation may cause myocardial ischemia; air typically embolizes to the right coronary artery causing transient ST elevation in the II, III, aVF ECG leads, hypotension and/or bradycardia. If air embolizes to the cerebral circulation it can cause a transient ischemic attack or a stroke that may not be recognized while the patient is under general anesthesia.

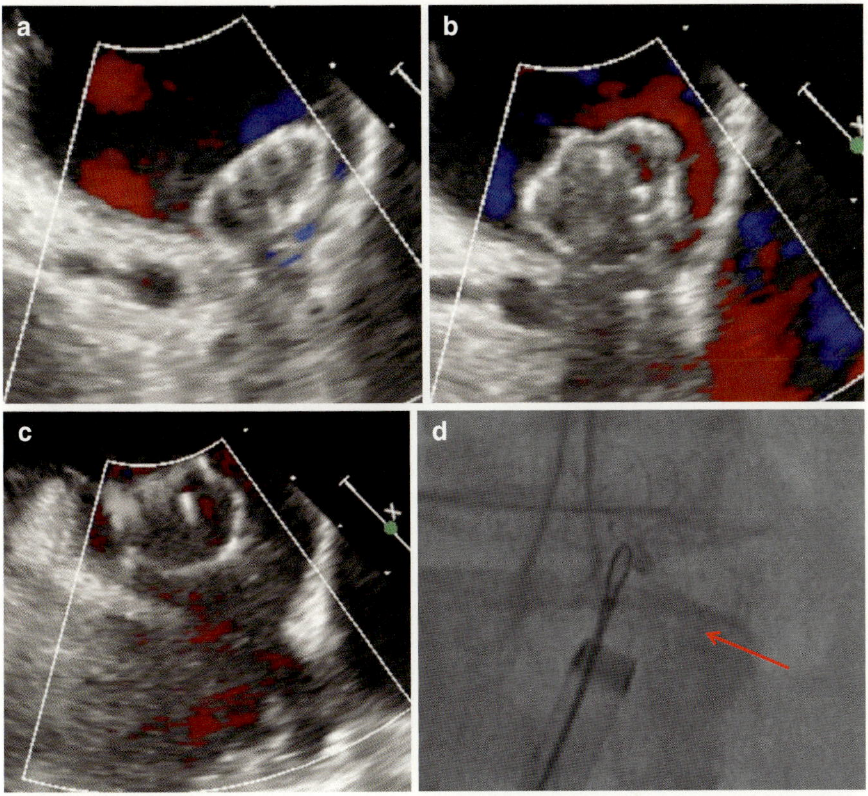

Fig. 9.12 *Watchman device embolization*. With a slightly different TEE view a larger than anticipated protrusion into the LA is seen (**a**). Shortly after this image and with the patient's in sinus rhythm constantly changing the LAA size the device becomes free (**b**, **c**). It immediately embolizes to the distal aorta (**d**). A 16F TAVI sheath (Cook) and a 30 mm snare are used to grab the 24 device somewhere near the knob. The device could not be removed through the sheath but had to be taken out anchored at the distal part of the sheath. The arterial puncture site was closed with the two ProGlide implanted prior to introducing the 16F sheath ("TAVI technique")

9.1.4.1 Prevention

- Maintenance of left atrial pressure > 10 mmHg (by administering 1 l of saline i.v.) is an important safety measure to prevent air embolism and is recommended by most operators.
- Meticulous flushing all catheters and careful device preparation is mandatory. In case there is a doubt about potential presence of air in the device, backbleeding is recommended. A last flush with contrast and a brief check under fluoroscopy can be helpful.

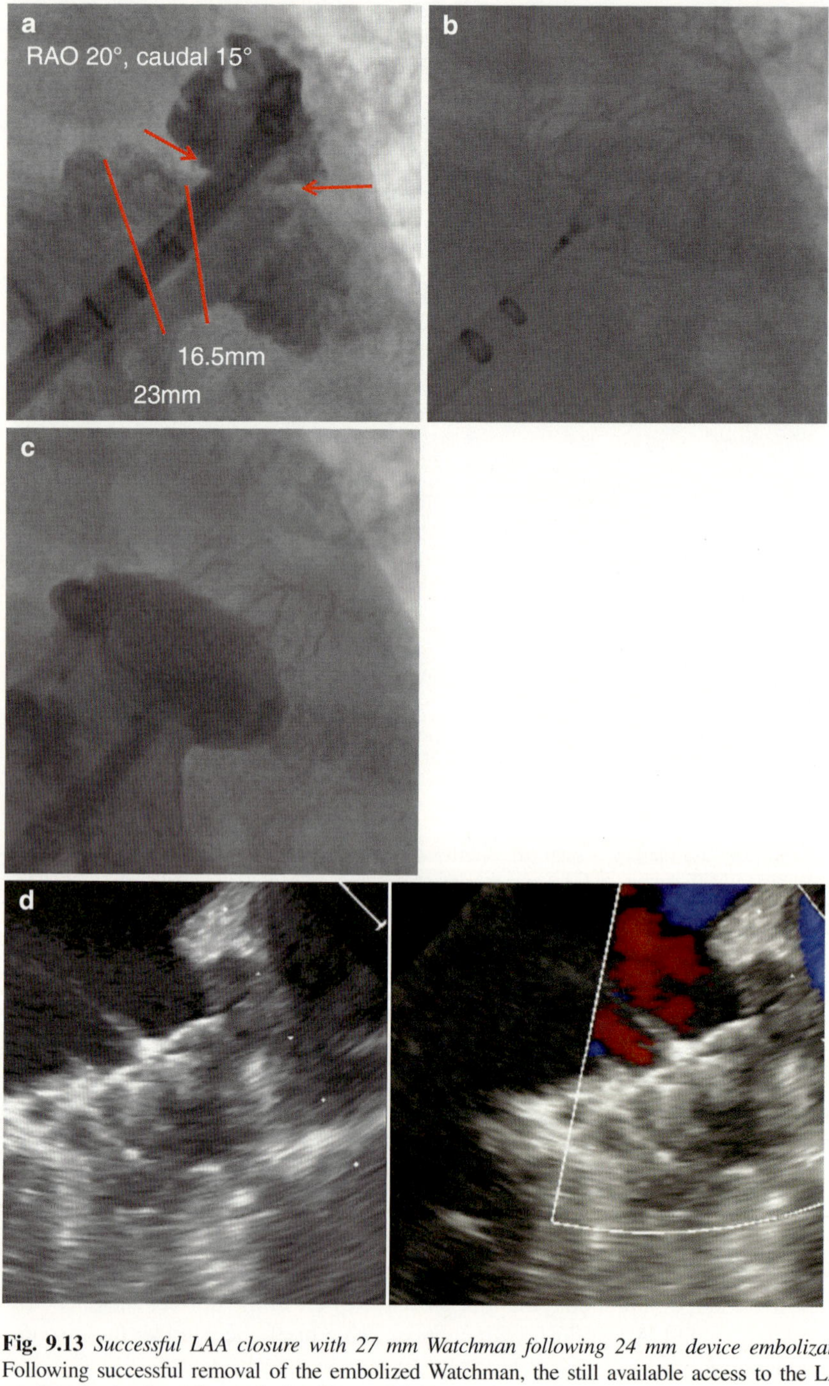

Fig. 9.13 *Successful LAA closure with 27 mm Watchman following 24 mm device embolization.* Following successful removal of the embolized Watchman, the still available access to the LA is employed to implant a larger device (27 mm Watchman) in a different position. (**a**) Initial LAA visualization, two sizing measurements are shown. (**b**) following release, the 27 mm device unfolds characteristically. (**c, d**). Angiography and echocardiography documents complete closure of the LAA

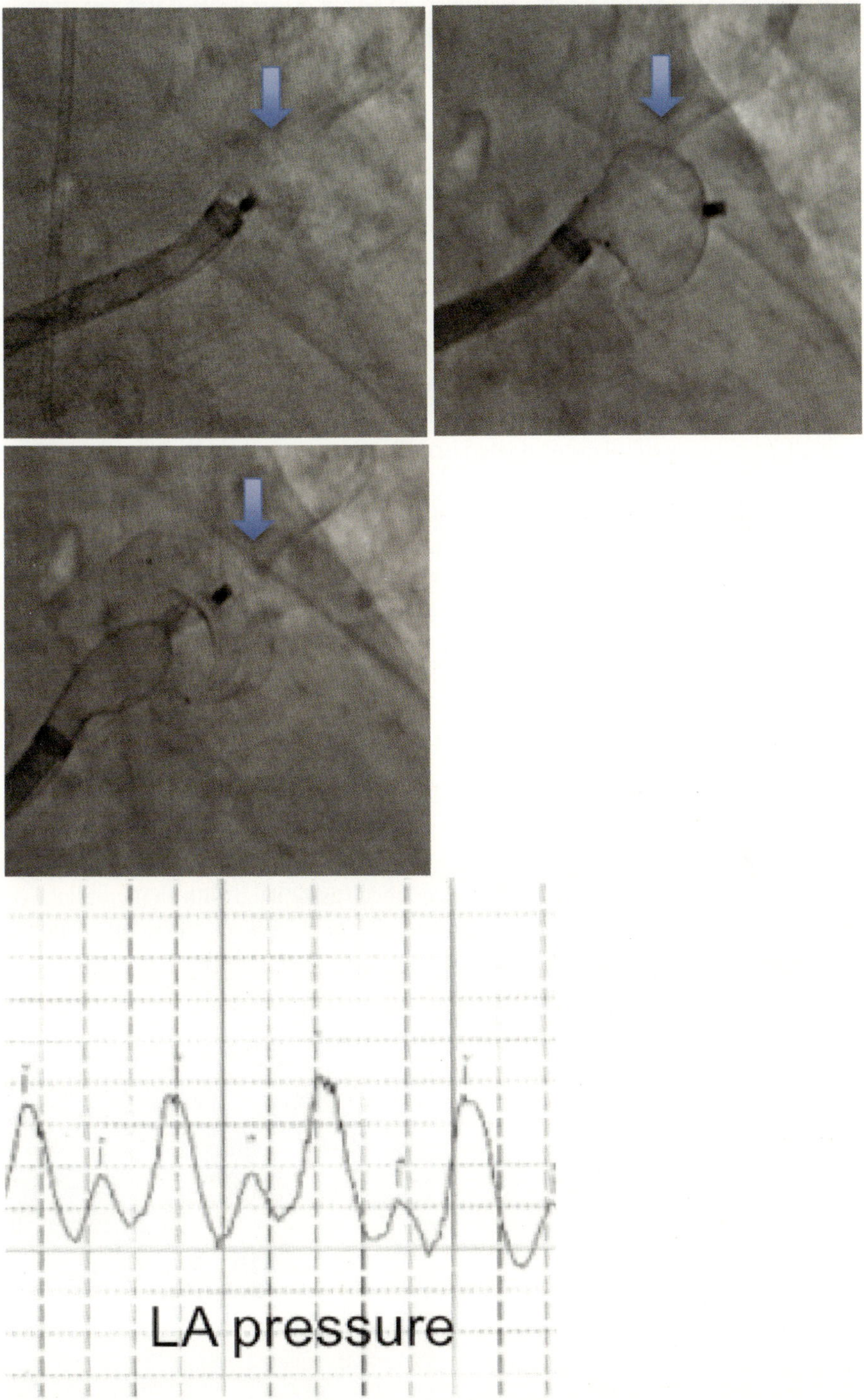

Fig. 9.14 Air embolism may occur during the procedure due to inadequate flushing or backbleeding of catheters or sheaths. Administration of 100% oxygen may prevent cerebral or myocardial ischemia. Maintaining the LA pressure >10 mmHg can prevent air aspiration during the procedure

- It should be noted that air in a sheath could be almost invisible if it is mixed with saline or blood. Preparatory filling the sheath with a small amount of contrast may help to reveal any air bubbles during device introduction. If this occurs, the safest way to clean the sheath is to remove the device completely, flush and reintroduce it in the sheath. Allowing just back-flow bleeding may remove part or all of the air but in the absence of contrast in the sheath, complete de-airing cannot be confirmed.
- General anesthesia with paralysis may also be protective, as the patient does not breath spontaneously so the thoracic pressure remains positive throughout.

9.1.4.2 Treatment

- The anatomy of the LAA, which is usually oriented upwards, may result in air entrapment within it. Air can be aspirated by using a large bore catheter. Device implantation maybe also considered in order trap the air, provided that the patient remains in supine position with added oxygen for a few hours.
- In case of anticipated or actual air embolism in the left heart circulation, administration of 100% oxygen can help reducing the ischemic damage to the heart or the brain. Usually small amounts of air are well tolerated and the patient recovers within a few minutes. In case of larger air emboli, more aggressive measures may be needed, starting with a selective angiogram and continuing with administration of nitrates, warm saline, etc.

9.1.5 Device Thrombosis During Follow Up

Device thrombosis is the most common complication at follow-up occurring in 3–4% of patients (Fig. 9.15). So far, it has not been associated with an increased risk for stroke. However, device thrombosis should be avoided and if it occurs it should be treated appropriately.

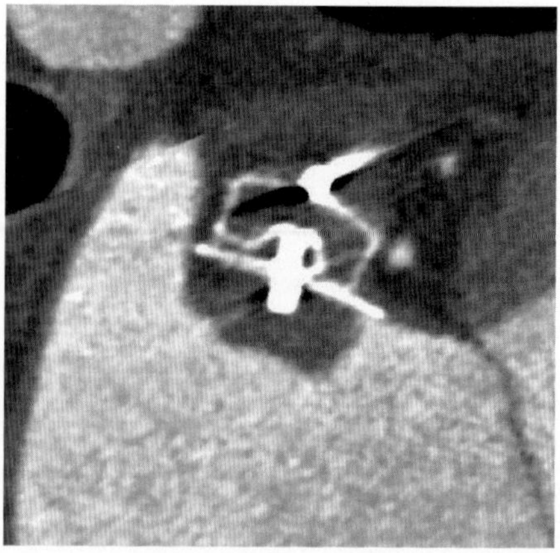

Fig. 9.15 Device thrombosis on the Amplatzer Cardiac Plug occurs at a rate of 2–20% in various published series

9.1.5.1 Prevention

- Administration of antithrombotic medication (antiplatelets or OAC) immediately after the procedure.
- Avoid leaving parts of the LAA uncovered due to overly deep or undersized device implantation.

9.1.5.2 Treatment

- Treatment with weight adjusted, high dose low molecular weight heparin (i.e. 2 × 0.8 mg clexane/day) or warfarin INR 2.5–3.0 typically leads to disappearance of the thrombus within 4–6 weeks (Fig. 9.16).
- Following thrombus resolution, dual antiplatelet is usually effective to prevent thrombus reappearing.

9.1.6 Late Pericardial Effusion/Tamponade

Late (>48 h post-procedure) pericardial effusion/tamponade is a rare (<1%) complication of LAA closure. In the recent prospective Watchman EWOLUTION registry, only two patients developed a late effusion.

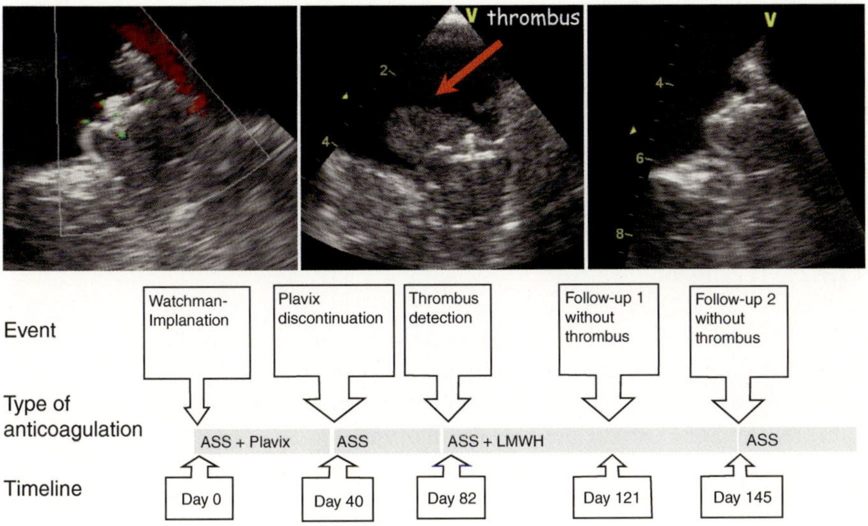

Fig. 9.16 Device thrombosis occurs at a rate of 3–5% on the Watchman device in large series. Here: Resolution of thrombus on a Watchman device. Dual anitplatelet therapy was stopped in this patient at day 40 contrary to the implanters recommendation. TEE at day 82 revealed a thrombus on the inferior part of the device; most thrombi on a Watchman device occur at this location. The patients was started on 2 × 0.6 mg enoxoparin s.c. for 40 days. Control TEE at day 145 revealed complete thrombus resolution without any neurologic events

9.1.6.1 Prevention

- In case of a pericardial effusion at baseline, the TEE or TTE follow-up should be more frequent, i.e. initially every month for the first 2–3 months and then every 3 months for the first year.
- Patients should be informed about this complication and should be notified that in case of unexplained hypotension they need to be examined by a physician.

9.1.6.2 Treatment

- Asymptomatic pericardial effusion is treated conservatively, either with anti-inflammatory drugs or colchicine or without medication and only frequent surveillance.
- Symptomatic pericardial effusion or cardiac tamponade is treated by pericardiocenteces.

9.1.7 Device Embolization

Late device embolization is rare and is caused by the same factors as for procedural device embolization [8]. It is usually asymptomatic, especially if the embolized device has crossed the aortic valve and is found in a peripheral vessel. No late embolization was observed with the Watchman device in the EWOLUTION registry following 1024 patients at the one year time point.

9.1.7.1 Prevention

- The same preventive measures as for acute device embolization apply.

9.1.7.2 Treatment

- Retrieval of a device that has embolized is performed in the same way as described for procedural embolizations. However, it should be noted that device endotheliazation and local attachment in the surrounding tissues may complicate the retrieval of a chronic peripheral embolization.

Acknowledgment The author would like to thank Kevin P. Walsh, Mater Misericordiae University Hospital, Dublin, Ireland for critical reading and helpful comments.

References

1. Park JW, Bethencourt A, Sievert H, et al. Left atrial appendage closure with Amplatzer cardiac plug in atrial fibrillation: initial European experience. Catheter Cardiovasc Interv. 2011;77:700–6.
2. Holmes DR, Reddy VY, Turi ZG, et al. Percutaneous closure of the left atrial appendage versus warfarin therapy for prevention of stroke in patients with atrial fibrillation: a randomised non-inferiority trial. Lancet. 2009;374:534–42.
3. Reddy VY, Doshi SK, Sievert H, et al. Percutaneous left atrial appendage closure for stroke prophylaxis in patients with atrial fibrillation: 2.3-year follow-up of the PROTECT AF (Watchman left atrial appendage system for embolic protection in patients with atrial fibrillation) trial. Circulation. 2013;127:720–9.
4. Reddy VY, Holmes D, Doshi SK, Neuzil P, Kar S. Safety of percutaneous left atrial appendage closure: results from the Watchman left atrial appendage system for embolic protection in patients with AF (PROTECT AF) clinical trial and the continued access registry. Circulation. 2011;123:417–24.
5. Tzikas A, Shakir S, Gafoor S, et al. Left atrial appendage occlusion for stroke prevention in atrial fibrillation: multicentre experience with the AMPLATZER Cardiac Plug. EuroIntervention. 2015;10
6. Main ML, Fan D, Reddy VY, et al. Assessment of device-related thrombus and associated clinical outcomes with the WATCHMAN left atrial appendage closure device for embolic protection in patients with atrial fibrillation (from the PROTECT-AF trial). Am J Cardiol. 2016;117:1127–34.
7. Tzikas A, Holmes Jr DR, Gafoor S, et al. Percutaneous left atrial appendage occlusion: the Munich consensus document on definitions, endpoints and data collection requirements for clinical studies. EuroIntervention. 2016;12:103–11.
8. Aminian A, Lalmand J, Tzikas A, Budts W, Benit E, Kefer J. Embolization of left atrial appendage closure devices: a systematic review of cases reported with the Watchman device and the Amplatzer cardiac plug. Catheter Cardiovasc Interv. 2015;86:128–35.

Chapter 10
Combined Procedures

10.1 LAA Closure and Transcatheter Aortic Valve Implantation (TAVI)

Episodes of atrial fibrillation are frequently observed after a TAVI procedure most likely linked to the altered hemodynamic situation after the reduction of the trans-aortic gradient and with LV hypertrophy being present in almost all patients. This is associated with an increased risk of stroke during follow. In addition, many octogenarians with an increased bleeding risk receive a TAVI. LAA closure as part of the initial procedure may therefore be beneficial in selected patients in order to prevent fatal bleedings. This combination of procedures has been performed both in routine as well as in several live cases at various international meetings, i.e. at EuroPCR and TCT [1]. Aside from patient's comfort of having only one procedure no particular benefit of combining both procedures could be demonstrated so far [2].

Most operators perform a TAVI procedure first by using a standard femoral access and then move on to occlude the LAA via a transvenous approach and transseptal puncture with the device they are most familiar with (Watchman or Amulet) thus avoiding prolonged procedure times. A TEE is not part of the TAVI procedure in many centers. Conscious sedation is sufficient for most TAVI procedures.

LAA closure can be performed through the femoral venous access that many centers use during a TAVI for the pacemaker lead or as a preventive measure if circulatory support is necessary. The TAVI prosthesis marks the aortic annulus which may serve as a landmark for transeptal puncture. LAA closure is performed following the usual standards. Post-implantation anticoagulation during the three months of device endothelialization may be done with either dual antiplatelet therapy or NOAC therapy-a therapeutic concept that is increasingly being used in this setting. NOAC's appear to have the same bleeding risk as dual antiplatelet therapy but the advantage of a much shorter half-life (EWOLUTION). There is no indication for triple therapy in this setting.

M.W. Bergmann et al., *Clinical Cases in LAA Occlusion*,
DOI 10.1007/978-3-319-51431-4_10

10.2 LAA Closure and MitraClip Implantation

Atrial fibrillation requiring stroke protection is also common in patients with mitral regurgitation. When a MitraClip implantation is chosen as therapeutic option to treat relevant mitral regurgitation in these patients, LAA closure during the same procedure seems to be attractive especially if an increased bleeding risk is present as the same access way can be used for the placement of both devices. However, there are two issues that question this approach: First, the implantation of a MitraClip usually leaves an increased gradient across the mitral valve behind that may increase the risk of thrombus formation in the free left atrial cavum rather than the LAA. Therefore the benefit of LAA closure in the setting of a MitraClip implantation may be limited. Secondly, for a MitraClip procedure the transseptal puncture site needs to be high above the mitral valve plane whereas LAA closure is easier with a low puncture site, particularly when an Amulet device is chosen [3] (around 4–4.5 cm vs. 3–4 cm above the mitral plane).

Most operators favor the concept to first finish the more complex MitraClip procedure and then move on to LAA closure [3, 4]. The TEE probe stays in place. Procedure time should be limited so operators should use the device they are familiar with. In case of Watchman LAA closure, the Watchman sheath is not long enough to be placed via the MitraClip sheath. A technique has been developed to employ a Proglide closure system that allows to exchange the Clip system for the LAA closure sheath through the same venous and transseptal access: the Proglide is only tightened to 50% in the first step and completely closed after removal of the LAA system. The Amplatzer system may be used via the MitraClip sheath.

Following successful MitraClip and LAA closure patients should receive oral anticoagulation using NOAC's for 3 months if possible in relation to the bleeding risk; alternatively dual antiplatelet therapy has been used. Longterm therapy is currently unclear and may depend on the transvalvular gradient after MitraClip implantation: if the gradient is increased (above 5 mmHg mean), oral anticoagulation may be necessary since the rate of thrombus from the left atrium not originating from the LAA will be significantly higher—in the setting of mitral stenosis, around 50% of thrombi originate not from the LAA.

10.3 LAA Closure and Percutaneous Coronary Interventions (PCI)

Following elective PCI with implantation of a drug-eluting stent (DES) 3–6 months dual antiplatelet therapy is necessary to prevent stent thrombosis. With the latest generation of DES one month of dual antiplatelet therapy (DPT) with clopidogrel and aspirin in combination seems to be acceptable in patients at high bleeding risk. The situation is completely different in patients following an acute coronary syndrome: at least one year of aggressive DPT combining ticagrelor or prasugrel with aspirin is recommended by current guidelines. Recent studies also see reduced cardiovascular events if DPT is prolonged to three years. In case of atrial fibrillation as a comorbidity, the issue of triple therapy arises. Triple therapy is not recommended as it is associated with an extremely increased, life threating bleeding risk. Aspirin can be omitted from the combination therapy, the 2016 guidelines on atrial fibrillation now recommend the combination of NOAC or warfarin with clopidogrel. No increased stent thrombosis has been observed with this combination; bleeding risk is reduced significantly.

Combining PCI with LAA closure mostly performed in a separate procedure has the advantage of dual antiplatelet therapy with ticagrelor or prasugrel combined with aspirin to be effective and sufficient for the prevention of both stroke and stent thrombosis. Especially in the setting of multivessel disease with expected further episodes of acute coronary syndromes, LAA closure allows to focus antithrombotic therapy on platelet inhibition [1]. This should be considered in all patients that receive PCI in the presence of atrial fibrillation. Studies are underway to explore this approach.

10.4 LAA Closure and Pulmonary Vein Isolation (PVI)

Patients with symptomatic atrial fibrillation (AF) should receive pulmonary vein isolation (PVI) if antiarrhythmic therapy is not successful; one may even consider PVI a first line therapy in young patients with paroxysmal atrial fibrillation [5]. PVI is more successful if performed early on in the disease course than if persistent AF is present. With the exception of lone atrial fibrillation in younger patients, stroke prevention is still necessary even if PVI restored sinus rhythm- the asymptomatic recurrence of AF is frequent. PVI does not reduce the risk of stroke; only patients with a CHA2DS2-VASc of ≤ 1 may consider to stop oral anticoagulation if no new episodes of AF occur after PVI. It is therefore reasonable to combine PVI with LAA closure. Technically the procedure can be performed easily by using the same transseptal puncture site as described in the EWOLUTION registry (Late breaking trial presentation at EuroPace 2016). The inferior ridge of the left superior pulmonary vein is anatomically in close proximity to the LAA ostium; the Watchman device is positioned distally to this area and is therefore first choice in this setting. Anticoagulation is performed according to local standards and the individual bleeding risk of the patient; transient NOAC therapy may be considered first choice.

References

1. Taramasso M, Maisano F, Nietlispach F. TAVI and concomitant procedures: from PCI to LAA closure. EuroIntervention. 2015;11(Suppl W):W96–100.
2. Bogunovic N, Scholtz W, Prinz C, Faber L, Horstkotte D, van Buuren F. Percutaneous closure of left atrial appendage after transcatheter aortic valve implantation—an interventional approach to avoid anticoagulation therapy in elderly patients: TAVI and closure of LAA to avoid warfarin therapy. EuroIntervention. 2012;7(11):1361–3.

3. Tichelbacker T, Puls M, Jacobshagen C, et al. MitraClip(R) and Amplatzer(R) cardiac plug implantation in a single procedure: a reasonable approach? Int J Cardiol. 2016;220:107–11.
4. Schade A, Kerber S, Hamm K. Two in a single procedure: combined approach for MitraClip implantation and left atrial appendage occlusion using the Watchman device. J Invasive Cardiol. 2014;26(3):E32–4.
5. Romanov A, Pokushalov E, Artemenko S, et al. Does left atrial appendage closure improve the success of pulmonary vein isolation? Results of a randomized clinical trial. J Interv Card Electrophysiol. 2015;44(1):9–16.

Index

M.W. Bergmann et al., *Clinical Cases in LAA Occlusion*,
DOI 10.1007/978-3-319-51431-4

Printed by Printforce, the Netherlands